The Quantum Wellness Cleanse

OTHER BOOKS BY KATHY FRESTON

The One: Discovering the Secrets of Soul Mate Love

Expect a Miracle: 7 Spiritual Steps to Finding the Right Relationship

Quantum Wellness: A Practical and Spiritual Guide to Health and Happiness

The Quantum Wellness Cleanse

THE 21-DAY ESSENTIAL GUIDE TO HEALING YOUR BODY, MIND, AND SPIRIT

Kathy Freston

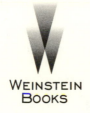

WEINSTEIN
BOOKS

ISBN-10: 1-6028-6091-2
ISBN-13: 978-1-6028-6091-9

First Edition
10 9 8 7 6 5 4 3 2 1

Contents

Foreword: 21 Days May Lead to a Lifetime of Pleasure and Feeling Good

PÈRE HENRI, THE PARISH PRIEST IN THE WONDERFUL MOVIE *Chocolat*, sums up the central message of the movie this way: "Listen, here's what I think. I think we can't go around measuring our goodness by what we *don't* do. By what we deny ourselves. What we resist, and who we exclude. I think we've got to measure goodness by what we embrace, what we create, and who we include."

What I like best about the book you have in your hands is that although its program involves making choices about what we consume on a regular basis, the larger framing of this book is an affirmation of pleasure and feeling good.

After more than thirty years of helping people change their lifestyles, I've learned what is sustainable: pleasure, abundance, and freedom—joy of living, not fear of dying. What you *include* in your diet is as important as what you *exclude*. And there's no point in giving up something that you enjoy unless you get something back that's even better—and quickly.

Life is to be fully enjoyed.

You have a spectrum of choices; it's not all or nothing. In our studies, we found that the more people changed, the better they felt and the more they improved. To the degree that you follow Kathy's recommendations in this book, you're likely to look better, feel better, lose weight, and gain health. Although the conventional wisdom has been that it's easier to make small changes in our lives than big ones, sometimes a comprehensive approach like the one outlined by Kathy in this book is more sustainable than an incremental one.

Why? Because big changes often cause considerable benefits, and more quickly than was once thought possible. You're likely to feel so much better, so quickly, that the reason for making these changes transforms from risk-factor reduction (which is boring), or fear of dying (which is too scary) to joy of living. You may find that what you reduce or give up is less important than what you gain.

The latest studies show how much more dynamic our bodies are than was previously believed. For example, there are minute-to-minute changes in how much blood flow different parts of your body receive. What you eat, and what you do, can increase or decrease this blood flow very quickly, with powerful effects—for better and for worse.

When you eat a healthier diet, quit smoking, exercise, meditate, and have more love in your life, then your brain receives more blood and oxygen, so you think more clearly, have more energy, need less sleep. Your brain may actually grow so many brain cells (neurons) that it gets measurably bigger in only three months. Your face gets more blood flow, so your skin glows more and wrinkles less. Your heart gets more blood flow, so you have more stamina and can even begin to reverse heart disease. Your sexual organs receive more blood flow, so you may become more potent—the same way that drugs like Viagra, Cialis, and Levitra work. For many people, these are choices worth making—not just to live longer, but also to live better.

In contrast, meals high in fat, sugar, and calories cause your arteries to constrict, so blood flow is reduced. So does chronic stress. So does nicotine in cigarettes. So do stimulants such as caffeine, cocaine, and amphetamines. So does a lack of exercise. How do you feel after you've just finished a holiday feast? Sleepy, like you want to take a nap.

Why? Because your brain is receiving less blood flow and oxygen. So is your skin, so you look older. So is your heart, so you may have less stamina. So are your sexual organs, and this interferes with your sexual potency.

Having seen what a powerful difference comprehensive lifestyle changes can make, I was happy to write this foreword. The author, Kathy Freston, has years of experience inspiring people to make intensive changes in diet and lifestyle that have helped transform their lives for the better. Her wisdom is distilled into the program outlined in this book.

Kathy's approach is multidimensional and multifactorial, a powerful blend of what works and why. It's not just about living longer, but also about living better—to help people find wellness: psychological happiness, physical health and vitality, and good relationships with ourselves and others. She addresses the underlying causes of many chronic illnesses rather than just literally or figuratively bypassing them. If we treat only the symptoms without also addressing their underlying causes, it's a little like mopping up the floor around a sink that's overflowing without turning off the faucet. The same problem comes back; or we get a new set of problems; or we have painful choices.

The need has never been more urgent:

- **More than 45 million Americans are currently without health insurance. At the time of this writing, President Obama is committed to addressing this important issue. Those of us consulting with his health reform team understand that if we are going to provide health insurance to those who don't have it without also changing the health care system to emphasize prevention and public health to reduce costs, then medical expenditures will increase substantially at a time when we can least afford it. But if we can treat the more fundamental causes of why people get sick, as Kathy's book addresses, our studies and those of others are showing that the body has a remarkable capacity to begin healing itself, and much more quickly than we had once realized, if we address the lifestyle factors that often cause these chronic diseases. These approaches are both medically effective and cost effective, thereby improving quality while reducing costs.**
- **Health care costs—really, disease care costs— often exceed net revenues for many corpora-**

tions. Heart disease, diabetes, prostate cancer, breast cancer, and obesity account for 75 percent of health care costs, and yet these are largely preventable and even reversible through changes in diet and lifestyle.

- The limitations of high-tech medicine are becoming more apparent. Recently, for example, more than 1.3 million coronary angioplasty procedures were performed at a cost of more than \$60 billion, and more than 450,000 coronary bypass operations were performed at a cost of another \$45 billion. Despite these costs, a recent randomized controlled trial published in *The New England Journal of Medicine* found that angioplasties and stents do not prolong life or even prevent heart attacks in stable patients (i.e., 95 percent of those who receive them). Coronary bypass surgery prolongs life in less than 3 percent of patients who receive it.

- The power of comprehensive lifestyle changes, such as those described in this book, is now well documented. The Interheart study, published in *The Lancet*, followed 30,000 men and women in six continents and found that lifestyle changes could prevent over 90 percent of heart disease. Thus, the disease that accounts for more premature deaths and costs more than any other illness is almost completely preventable. And the same lifestyle changes that can prevent or even reverse heart disease also help prevent or even reverse many other chronic diseases as well.

- In our randomized controlled trials, published in the *Journal of the American Medical Association*, *The Lancet*, and other major medical and scientific journals, my colleagues and I found that most people with severe coronary heart disease were able to stop or reverse it by making comprehensive lifestyle changes, without drugs or surgery. Most of the patients with severe angina (chest pain) became pain-free within only a few weeks, and their quality of life improved dramatically. We found that the progression of early prostate cancer can be stopped or even reversed through lifestyle change. Our newest studies, published in the *Proceedings of the National Academy of Sciences* and *The Lancet Oncology* found that lifestyle changes also alter hundreds of genes in only a few months, "turning on" disease-preventing genes and "turning off" genes that promote heart disease, breast cancer, prostate cancer, and other illnesses. We found that lifestyle changes significantly increase *telomerase*, the enzyme that repairs and lengthens *telomeres*, the ends of our chromosomes that control how long we live. As our telomeres get longer, so do our lives.

Fortunately, at a time when people are more confused than ever, there is an emerging consensus about what constitutes a healthy way of living. It looks a lot like what Kathy Freston recommends in this book.

Dean Ornish, M.D.
Founder and President,
Preventive Medicine Research Institute
Clinical Professor of Medicine,
University of California, San Francisco

FOREWORD

IN *THE QUANTUM WELLNESS CLEANSE*, KATHY FRESTON HITS US
right between the eyes.

I'm going to get several copies of this book and put them
in different rooms in my house. It's not so much that it's a
"pick it up and read it anywhere" kind of book, as that it's
information that, while very simple, leads to radically different behavioral patterns from the ones I adhere to now. I
keep reading certain things over and over again, experiencing the trickle-down of information from my intellect to
my gut.

We all know by now Margaret Mead's famous saying that
we should never doubt that a small group of concerned citizens can change the world; in fact, it's the only thing that
ever has. She is talking about social revolution: how one set
of ideas gives way to another. Today we are living at a time
of profound social revolution—indeed several of them are
going on at once. And one of them—in Freston's opinion,
fundamental to them all—is a revolution in how we view

food. We are awakening to a connection between food and consciousness that is new to the Western world, and the awakening is reaching a tipping point that is starting to affect us all.

Margaret Mead was right to point out the power of small groups, but there is another issue, one she didn't address in her famous quote: the role that individuals often play in harnessing the power of the small group. Kathy Freston has made a beautiful mosaic out of movements that have been growing for years. She has taken subjects ranging from vegetarianism to concern for the treatment of animals to spiritual enlightenment and woven them into an elegant package of contemporary understanding. She has created a unique and powerful platform for lifting our thoughts and behavior to a higher plane, and she has done all this in a way that makes it seem easy. She has sauntered into our popular imagination and, with a wave of her most lovely hand, led a revolution in a major area of our thinking. Wherever you are with your food, your consciousness about animals, or your spiritual practice, reading this book is going to take you to a higher place.

There's an interesting thing about popularizers, those people who can take a serious, complicated subject and make it accessible to the masses. While their work is easy (and convenient) for specialists to denigrate, the truth is that a powerful popularizer cannot do what he or she does—cannot move masses of people—unless she herself understands the deeper substance of her subject. The world has Nobel Prize winners in all the subjects Freston discusses in this book— from biodiversity to forgiveness, from the biology of digestion to the practice of meditation—but it took Kathy Freston to put these things together in the reasonable, intelligent, and doable twenty-one-day plan that you are holding in your hands right now.

We're a generation that has been transitioning for a while now, from just yearning for things to yearning for meaning. We want to be conscious citizens in a world that is clearly in peril; we want to help shift the trajectory of human history from the probability of disaster to the possibility of a miracle. We want to be strong enough to become leaders, and humble enough to be followers when true leaders show up in our midst. Kathy Freston is not only a writer; she is a leader. She leads us to greater understanding of our bodies, our minds, our fellow creatures, our planet, and our spirits; and like all true leaders, she leads us beyond simple understanding to actual practice. In this book, you'll find more than mere information; you'll find practical guidance for how to use that information to become a better, more effective, more conscious human being.

In *The Quantum Wellness Cleanse,* Freston covers an amazing array of subjects with intelligence and grace. Give her the twenty-one days she asks for, and you'll see the world around you differently. In ways both big and small, this book has the power to change your life.

—Marianne Williamson

INTRODUCTION

I RECENTLY PUBLISHED MY THIRD BOOK, *QUANTUM WELLNESS: A Practical and Spiritual Guide to Health and Happiness.* That book details how small, incremental changes—in what we eat, how we think, how we move our bodies, and how we relate to others—can reap huge rewards. One of the practices I recommend for "jump-starting" a quantum shift to a higher state of wellness is a 21-Day Cleanse—a period of three weeks in which you abstain from sugar, caffeine, gluten, alcohol, and animal products, and load yourself full of a wholesome, plant-based diet. Of all the things I wrote about in that book, it was the cleanse that elicited the most overwhelming response. Easily 90 percent of the questions and letters I receive from readers have to do with navigating those twenty-one days. Clearly, a nerve has been struck. I don't think it's just that people want to detox and lose weight, although that is surely part of it. I think that the promise of experiencing real, discernible breakthroughs in body, mind, and spirit in a relatively short period of time appeals to the great many of us who have a serious desire for personal development and change.

And so I decided to devote a whole book to the cleanse—to answering your questions, going into greater depth about the process, and offering you a hand as you try to go three weeks without some of the substances you reach for when you need comfort. Get ready for a miracle, because that's what happens when you first make the decision to move in the direction of quantum wellness, when you decide to take supremely good care of your body and work through the obstacles that come up when you do. When you make your move—even if it's a just a single step—toward the shift you'd like to experience, your body, mind, and spirit are brought to a whole new and altogether higher level.

I started doing cleanses more than twenty-five years ago because I wanted to lose weight, plain and simple. I hoped that taking a little break from my (over)eating routine might snap me out of unhealthy patterns. I started off by fasting every Monday, forgoing all food except a mixture of apple cider vinegar, honey, and water. After a while, I moved on to juice fasts, where for a few days or even a week at a time I would consume only juices made from fruits, carrots, spinach, celery, ginger, and other vegetables. At other times over the years I tried the various programs that were in vogue and that promised some sort of miracle. What I found was that fasting didn't work for me. I never experienced the promised weight loss or, if I did, it didn't last. In fact, whenever I would fast, my metabolism would slow way down and put my body on starvation alert. In other words, whatever calories

I *did* ingest, my body would hang on to tightly because it wasn't so sure that more would be coming in.

For many people, these practices have their merits, and many are quite detoxifying and healing, but they didn't work for me. Plus, not eating made me anxious and I couldn't concentrate; all I could think about was what I would eat for that first "break-fast" meal.

The Quantum Wellness 21-Day Cleanse is nothing like those punishing fasts I tried. It is extremely simple and nutritionally sound. In fact, it is more a healthy way of living than it is a harsh or difficult discipline. It's about choosing foods that don't tax the body and make it work so hard; it's about taking a break but not about starving.

The more I studied and looked into the ancient practice of giving up certain foods for a designated period of time, the more I realized that fasting and cleansing are not only good for making physical improvements, but they can also be a pathway to greater clarity and even enlightenment. Many masters throughout the ages have forgone food for periods of time so that they might feel closer to Spirit and less attached to the pedestrian rites of this world. They would give up a number of things—perhaps just taking in the bare essentials—and go into a deep meditation or discourse with a teacher. Or, like Gandhi, they would give up eating as a way of making a strong and committed statement that would bring about changes in social conditions and a shift toward higher societal consciousness.

The more I learned about fasting and cleansing traditions, the more I saw the wisdom in giving my body an occasional retreat so that I could break free from some of my lesser habits and cravings and the impulse for immediate gratification. From the early founders of Western medicine—Hippocrates, Galen, and Paracelsus—I learned that occasionally refraining from food was also a proven way to prevent and even cure disease. Even the great philosophers Plato, Socrates, and Pythagoras regularly gave up food (or certain foods) so that they could enhance and enliven their sense of physical well-being.

This cleanse is so simple and so powerful. For three weeks, you will refrain from eating what I call the "Big Five":

- **caffeine**
- **alcohol**
- **gluten**
- **animal products**
- **sugar**

On first glance, it may seem like there will be nothing left to eat or drink! In fact, you will discover that there is a whole world of delicious and nutritious food to enjoy that will help you feel more energetic, healthy, and clean. And I guarantee you will not be hungry (unless you forget to eat!). This is a "diet" you could stay on indefinitely, because it doesn't deny your body any of its needs and is actually rich in nutritious vegetables, whole grains, fruits, and nuts, and chock-full of everything you need to fuel your body for a lifetime.

Over the course of the three weeks you'll be reading in some depth about why you're avoiding these Big Five categories, but for now just trust me when I say that these substances are difficult for our bodies and can even be toxic, and that a break from them will do you a world of good. We won't be doing any calorie counting or maniacally restricting carbs; I'll just be here to remind you to eat lots of grains, beans, nuts, seeds, fruits, and vegetables—which are loaded with naturally occurring vitamins and minerals—and give you plenty of suggestions for how to make them a part of your diet. Simple, no?

I want to prepare you for the physiological downside that some people experience for a few days. Many people experience no physical problems or actual signs of withdrawal, but some people do: if you are in the latter category, please remind yourself that this is a signal of addiction, and you don't want to be addicted. Please also keep reminding yourself that these bad physical feelings pass within a few days for almost everyone.

I know when I give up caffeine I get cranky and lethargic for the first few days. But that's part of the point. I become aware of just how dependent my body has become on an artificial boost and how it has forgotten how to feel good on its own. Some people get headaches when they kick caffeine, but these pass within a few days at the most.

Sugar can be another hard one for some people, especially people who are used to multiple sugary sodas or snacks every single day. But, as you probably know all too well, the sugar high is short-lived and often exacts a heavy price. We need more and more to feel the lift, and no matter how much we ingest, we never feel great (and all the while we're gaining weight from the calories and unused glycogen). In fact, we often feel downright spun out and desperate for the next fix—

almost like a drug addict. In a few pages, we'll look at why it's so important to purge processed sugars from your diet, at least for a short time. I'll also give you suggestions for alternative sweets.

If you are a steady drinker and you give up alcohol, you will likely experience the stress and anxiety that you were trying to blot out with the wine or vodka or what have you. My advice is to take this opportunity to gently and with great compassion for yourself face the very things you've been running from and maybe think about dealing with them in a whole new way. If an old trauma is weighing on you, you might want to check out a support or fellowship group; learn to meditate and exercise to renew the feel-good chemicals— dopamine, serotonin, and endorphins—that your brain naturally produces. As you learn to face your demons, whatever they may be, you will see that they are not as omnipotent as you thought they were. (However, if your relationship with alcohol is at all problematic for you I urge you to get support.) You will tap into an inner reserve of serenity (I will help you along the way) while finding that you are part of something larger that wants your healing to occur. This "flow" of healing energy will make itself known if you want it to.

Even if you are only a social drinker (like me), not having a drink with friends at a festive dinner can be challenging. You want to fit in and enjoy yourself just like everyone else; but this discomfort will be short-lived as you realize you don't need alcohol to relax and feel at ease. The more present you are to the conversation, the less you will crave the comfort of a drink. Changing our habits is shaky business at first, as habits come about because they provide some sense of security and regularity in the face of anxiety. But the more you lean in to the discomfort, instead of running from it or grabbing another drink, as long as you have a willingness to breathe through the difficult feelings, you will become more and more free to live at the highest levels of wellness.

As you read on about how an alcoholic drink is metabolized, you will see that it acts a lot like sugar in the body; you might get intense cravings and feel agitated if you don't "get your fix." Of course, this is all the more reason to break the physical habituation, at least for the length of the cleanse.

Giving up gluten will not cause a physical sense of withdrawal, because you are likely to experience an almost instant relief from digestive problems (if you have them). The difficulty you may have, though, is in finding things that don't contain gluten. Breads and other products made with rice, corn, quinoa, potatoes, oats, and buckwheat are good bets. Honestly, just getting out of the bread habit alone will have you feeling leaner and cleaner in no time. Many people don't have an issue with gluten (I don't). But processed flours react in the body much the way straight sugar does. One of the more immediate benefits of giving up processed flours for this short time is that you put a pause on overindulging in the breads and cereals that tend to cause weight gain and fatigue.

Despite what you may have heard, abstention from animal products will not deprive your body of any essential nutrients, and you won't feel tired or weak. There are plenty of proteins and amino acids in plant-based food, without all the unhealthy fat and additives. However, if meat was the mainstay of your diet before, you might feel a little lost and left out. This is good. It shakes things up. In fact, giving up animal products is one of the most important gifts you can give your body, mind, and spirit. And I will walk you through it, helping you discover all the ways to eat without animal protein. You may be breaking from the crowd, but you will also, at least temporarily, find yourself leading the pack for more holistic and responsible living. More on that later.

While I want to warn you that you may have cravings, I also want to stress that there are many, many people who don't have a hard time at all, and also stress that almost everyone feels lighter and more energetic within a day or two—I hear from people constantly who say they didn't even realize that they could feel so good. Their lethargic way of being had become their constant; with the cleanse, they realized that they could have more energy, need less sleep, and feel lighter and clearer, just by breaking their reliance on foods that are not right for the human body.

Simply put, what you are doing in this cleanse is eliminating common craving triggers, which are notorious for perpetuating the munchies (and then the self-flagellation that follows), as well as other unconstructive eating habits. You are giving your body a break from artificial stimulants and depressants, and in so doing you will find your own natural balance. You are giving your body both a good detox and a chance to release itself from the vicious cycle of addictive eating or drinking and the shame that follows. These are some big changes to make, I know, but we will make them methodically, learning about each as we go. It may feel like a swirl of chaos as you find your way, but things will become clearer and easier sooner than you can imagine.

The body is a brilliant and masterful system of healing and rejuvenation; it can often restore itself to perfect health if given half a chance. And the cleanse is part of that push toward restoration. It will give your body a reprieve from old and tired ways so that you can gather your strength and then surge to a higher level of wellness.

Why twenty-one days? Because that's about how long it takes for your tastes and cravings to begin responding to healthier and simpler foods. So what you are left with after completion is a whole new and healthier routine, balanced blood sugar and freedom from old addictions.

There are so many reasons to do this cleanse. You may be motivated by a desire to trim a few pounds, or you may be doing it to detox from all the things you put in your body that you know are not the healthiest. Personally, I do it at least once a year simply to give myself an opportunity to reboot. We all have routines or habits around food that come to control us, and the cleanse gives us a chance to see these habits with clear eyes. I know that whenever I find myself thinking I "couldn't possibly" give up this or that, I realize just how much I am owned by it. If it's coffee that I think I can't live without, I know it's time to let go of coffee for a while and see what happens. If I've been turning to ice-cream sundaes to calm my anxiety, then it's ice-cream sundaes that I have to live without, at least for a short time, so I can remember that I am more powerful than the food.

Don't we all want to be free and strong and happy, rather than dragged through life by our petty attachments? A cleanse is a great place to start.

You see, the Quantum Wellness Cleanse is not just good for the body; it's also good for the soul. As you read the daily notes and pointers, you will learn how to eat in a humane and compassionate way, and how your choices play out in the environment. After three weeks you can expect to have lost a little bit of weight and have more energy, but most important, you will have found a way to eat that aligns you with your inner values of kindness and integrity. You will most certainly be a whole lot healthier in every respect.

Doing this cleanse is one of the best ways I know to discover any negative emotional material we are covering over with food, so that we can shake it right out of our system. And the beauty of it is that you can take what feels right from this program and leave the rest behind. Once you've done the work, you can add things back in, though many people find that they want to stick with the changes that have so improved the way they look and feel.

Some of the changes you can expect from the 21-Day Quantum Wellness Cleanse are:

- **more energy**
- **clearer skin and eyes**
- **weight loss**
- **cessation of certain aches, pains, and digestive ailments**
- **release from addictive habits**

- **a profound and deepened awareness of your personal power and the effect you have in the world**

Truly, it is a jump-start to a whole new level of living and being.

Here's the thing about wellness: it's a continuum. We get better at it as we go. We get more informed, build esteem, and find what works as we keep putting one foot in front of the other. We develop new tastes and discover different and interesting foods, and we move into a new rhythm. And with every day that we say, "Okay, I'm bigger than my old habits," we rise to our greater selves. We soar. Consider this cleanse a gift you can give yourself anytime you need it—a gift that will improve your overall wellness, not only by giving you the best possible nutrition but also by getting you to look at everything that comes up during the process: emotions, struggles, triumphs, new tools, and fresh ways of understanding how connected everything is.

You will discover how some of the foods from which you are abstaining have been affecting your body and your mental state. You'll discover some of your emotional attachments to conditioned ways of thinking; for instance, when you're unhappy, do you go for the cookies? Don't dismiss that as typical—it is, but it's also something that you can overcome if you want to, at least for twenty-one days, and you're likely to feel a deep sense of satisfaction when you do (and rightly so). And that may also spur you to take a closer look at where that attachment came from and whether it makes sense to hold on to it when the cleanse is over.

To this day, I do the cleanse with the full knowledge that doing so gives my body a break from its heavy workload, so that I can get rid of some old, stored-up junk and undertake some of my most important inner work—freeing myself from negative bonds and challenging myself to better understand my inner life and how it connects to all life. In this way, I not only heal myself, but I contribute to the healing of our precious world.

I encourage you to read through the book once to get a feel for the overall picture of the cleanse and then go back and take each day one at a time. We'll cover a lot of ground, but in increments. By the time you complete your first cleanse, you will know yourself so much better. You will find yourself relating to other people and the world around you in a more satisfying, more genuine way because you will be penetrating some of your own defenses, and you will find yourself, on the whole, much clearer about many things. Over the course of the twenty-one days, I will be encouraging you to think deeply about where your food comes from and how its handling and its journey to your plate affect how you feel in your body and affect the environment around you; that will naturally raise your empathy for what others go through, too. This not only tends to make you more connected on a personal level, it also makes for a friendlier world.

But best of all, you will be spending three weeks eating delicious, nutrient-dense, fiber-rich food. And you won't be hungry at all!

This cleanse has no strange concoctions to drink, no pills you must go out and purchase. And of course it's medically unassailable. Nevertheless, do consult with your doctor before beginning, as it's always wise to check in with your medical advisers. If you can, go to a doctor who is well versed in the latest peer-reviewed research on nutrition.

Remember, the cleanse is a jump start to having a healthier body, a clearer mind, and a deeper sense of conscious awareness. It's a way of setting into motion your own personal revolution so that you might contribute to an even broader revolution. You don't have to maintain it forever, however; that will be up to you. (You might want to check out www .drgreger.org/DVDs/ for a good overview of the recent scientific nutrition literature.)

People often ask me about "discipline." They worry that they won't be able to get through the cleanse or do it perfectly. Here's what I tell them: challenge yourself, but don't make yourself (or others around you) crazy. Do the best you can. If something, such as soy milk, has a tiny bit of sweetener in it and you can't find one that doesn't, enjoy it without worry. If it's your birthday or anniversary, have a glass of champagne (unless you think you are an alcoholic and this would become a slippery slope). If you are at someone's dinner party and they have absolutely nothing you can eat except the pasta and it's not gluten-free, have the pasta and then pick back up the next day. Our goal is progress, not perfection! This won't be a piece of cake (okay, pun intended), but it shouldn't be oh-so-difficult. The first few days will be the hardest, and then you will find your footing and off you'll go!

For many people, it's easier to do the cleanse with friends so you can check in with and support one another. Some people start blog groups so they can share recipes and fellowship. You might have a willing partner or spouse who is interested, or you may entice your entire office to join in, which always makes the cleanse a fun and interesting event. Often enough, though, you will be on your own, which is just fine, too!

And know this: even if you decide that it's just too difficult to give up the Big Five all at once, you can choose to abstain from just one or two of the substances and make that your cleanse. That's okay; next time around, maybe you'll try more. I would suggest starting off with eliminating animal products if you have to choose just one. But do challenge yourself to go beyond what's comfortable and see if you can't go full throttle!

However you go about doing the cleanse, the journey will be uniquely yours, and the changes you experience will be perfect and appropriate for you. Get inspiration from your peers, but trust that your soul knows *exactly* what it needs to progress and thrive. Listen to the wisdom that will whisper to you along the way, and may you realize the shift in your life that you always knew was possible.

GET READY

NOW THAT YOU KNOW THE BASICS OF WHAT TO EXPECT, YOU'RE going to spend the next three days doing a little advance work. You'll be taking a close look at where you are now, so that you can get a sense of what you most need to focus on during your cleanse.

We are all at different points along the continuum of wellness; we arrive at and handle different junctures according to our own personal comfort levels. We may be ahead of the game in physical fitness while lagging behind in spiritual awareness, or very emotionally and psychologically astute, but lazy in the way we eat. Wherever you are is okay. You don't even have to share it with anyone. Just be honest with yourself about where you are. Then you can see exactly where you need to work and grow.

Please ask yourself the following questions. And remember, there are no right or wrong answers.

As I think about starting this cleanse:

How do I feel, overall? Physically, emotionally, and spiritually?

What do I suspect needs to change?

Where will I come up against the most resistance?

Am I willing to stretch myself beyond my previous limits so that I break through the resistance?

Can I take in new information and let it settle into my awareness, thus letting it change me?

Am I forever bound to my old ways, or do I have it within me to finally move forward?

Now let's take things a little further.

For three days before beginning the cleanse, write in a journal about your current eating habits so that you can become more aware of what drives you. Write down everything you put into your body for breakfast, lunch, dinner, drinks, and snacks. Don't hold anything back, and don't try to regulate yourself more than usual. Note the time, the amount you consume, and, if you can, your mood immediately before, during, and after eating. The purpose of this is to familiarize yourself with your feelings and impulses, because the better you know yourself, the more adeptly you will be able to navigate the challenges that will present themselves in the days ahead.

Becoming mindful about food and eating is an essential

piece of the health puzzle, especially for emotional eaters. You may notice that when you feel sad, you tend to eat—or overeat—carbohydrates. Many people turn to sugar or caffeine when they are tired. Others go to fats when they feel anxiety. Once you start looking at how and why you eat the way you do, you may find that you use food to self-medicate (take yourself out of an uncomfortable emotional state) rather than just to nourish the body with what it actually wants or needs. We all do this to some extent, but the trick is to gradually become more conscious of our inner workings.

We can't change anything until we first have awareness; when something is unconscious, it cannot be shifted or changed because we don't even realize it's there. So be vigilant in your observations and don't hold back. Write down everything you ingest, and why. And please don't beat yourself up about any of this—the more honest and forgiving you are with yourself, the more you will be open to making changes.

After taking your three-day inventory, look over your pages and ask yourself the following questions:

- **Do I feel that what I regularly put into my body is serving me well in terms of my overall health?**

- **What are the habits I would like to change or upgrade?**

And that's it: pay attention, get to know yourself, listen to your inner voice. This cleanse gives you a new context within which you can heal and change. Instead of punishing your body by feeding it the wrong stuff, you can send yourself a little compassion, knowing that you are doing the best you can and that things are about to get better.

Now state your intention to use this cleanse to become healthier in body, mind, and spirit.

Upon completion of your three days of journaling, begin the cleanse. Read through each day, digesting the information slowly, without racing forward, and with an openness and willingness to take in new ideas. Do the exercises and meditations, try the tips. And get ready for a quantum leap!

Week One

Day 1:

Lean In

TODAY IS GOING TO BE TRICKY, NO DOUBT. PROBABLY YOUR MORN-
ing ritual has already been stood on its head. No coffee, no
muffin or bagel. What are you going to do?

Restock your cupboards.

Whenever I begin a cleanse, I like to spend part of the
first day at the grocery store, stocking up on all the delicious,
wholesome foods I will enjoy for the next few weeks. To make
it easy for you, I've drawn up a shopping list of items that you
can find at any standard grocery store, so your pantry and
fridge will be full of all the right foods for the first days of the
cleanse. If you've never been down the natural foods aisle in
your local supermarket or into a health food store, get ready
for an adventure. There's a whole world of incredibly delicious and wholesome food waiting for you there. Try a few
new items with each shopping trip. There will be some you
love and some you don't, but the only way to discover new
foods to love is by being willing to experiment a little.

I've listed some "quickie meals" at the back of the book

that will help you to formulate your daily menus. There are three weeks' worth of fantastic recipes listed as well, so look through them and pick out a few you'd like to start with. The following are some of the basics.

General Grocery List
- Irish steel-cut oats. Oats do contain some gluten, but for most people they are quite tolerable. Unless you are particularly sensitive, they are okay to use.
- Mixed-grain hot cereals. Be sure they're gluten- and sugar-free—and this means no honey or maple syrup.
- Rice cakes
- Flax crackers
- Gluten-free bread. There are many delicious alternatives. Try some sprouted breads, as they are easier to digest and are less processed. You can usually find wonderful options such as millet and rice bread in the freezer section of the store. Also, if you surf the Net, there is a whole host of selections you can order and have delivered to your home!
- Sweet potatoes, yams
- Grains: brown or wild rice, millet, quinoa, amaranth, buckwheat, corn. You can even find precooked brown rice on store shelves in vacuum-sealed packages or in the freezer case. Cook your own if you can, but these are also fine.

- Nuts: almonds, walnuts, cashews, soy nuts, macadamia nuts, filberts, etc.
- Seeds: sunflower, pumpkin, sesame, hemp, flax. Flaxseeds must be freshly ground rather than eaten whole, otherwise they will go straight through your body without giving you their full nutritional benefit.
- Nut or seed butters: almond butter, tahini, cashew butter, peanut butter (all unsweetened)
- Vegan butter
- Vegan mayonnaise
- Nondairy protein powder (soy, pea, hemp, or rice-based)
- Beans and legumes: black beans, lentils, chickpeas, lima beans, adzuki beans, black-eyed peas, edamame, fava beans. Dried beans are best, but they do take a while to cook. Canned are also fine.
- Tofu
- Tempeh
- Faux meats: burgers, sausage patties, "meat crumbles," "chicken" patties. Make sure all are gluten-free.
- Artichoke, rice, or quinoa pasta
- Pasta sauce
- Vegetables: kale, broccoli, cauliflower, green beans, asparagus, brussels sprouts, zucchini, eggplant, collard greens, squash (butternut, spaghetti, acorn), tomatoes, etc.

- Mushrooms: shiitake, hen of the woods, portobello. Grilled, they make a great centerpiece for a meal.
- Salad: arugula, radicchio, endive, mixed greens, peppers, avocado, tomato, radish, etc.
- Fruits: apples, cherries, peaches, blueberries, goji berries; frozen fruits for smoothies; lemons, limes, and unsweetened pomegranate juice for sparkling-water cocktails
- Herbal teas such as mint, chamomile, vanilla spice, etc.
- Nondairy milk, such as rice, almond, hemp, or soy milk (unsweetened)
- Sweeteners: xylitol, agave nectar, and stevia for smoothies, milks, cereals, baked goods, etc.; use sparingly.
- Extra-virgin olive oil, expeller-pressed organic canola, high-oleic versions of sunflower and safflower oils, walnut oil, and flaxseed oil (the last is good to pour over things like salad or baked yam, but not to cook with).
- Seasonings: garlic, ginger, tamari; Himalayan crystal or Celtic sea salt. Regular table salt is bleached and stripped of minerals.
- Flours to cook or bake with: bean, pea, soy, potato, buckwheat, tapioca, nut and seed, arrowroot, and rice. There are also prepackaged flour mixes that cater to the gluten-free shopper.
- Popcorn

- Corn chips
- Guacamole
- Hummus
- Soy cheese (rennet-free)
- Frozen spinach, broccoli, and cauliflower to throw into smoothies . . . you won't even taste it!
- Vegetarian stock for cooking

You see, when people ask you what's left to eat without animal products, alcohol, caffeine, gluten, and sugar, you can tell them there is plenty!

Try some prepared foods from health food stores. They are often very tasty and nutritious. Visit the deli/salad bar area, too. And as much as possible, try to buy organic foods to avoid dangerous pesticides, antibiotics, and herbicides.

When I'm on the cleanse I no longer think about the foods I *can't* eat. Instead I look forward to my favorite snacks. I get excited thinking about the big salad I will make for lunch. I'll throw everything under the sun in there and then top it with some crumbled veggie burger patties. If I'm hungry between meals, I eat some mixed nuts, tamari almonds, a nutrition bar, or a piece of fruit. I can't wait for dinner, when I get to dig into a luscious fajita with black beans and guacamole with salsa. Or maybe a hearty lentil soup with some flax crackers on the side. And I make sure to have a variety of vegetables or salad a few times a day.

Leaning in to Change

Because you are giving up a lot at once, you might feel some withdrawal symptoms, especially during the first few days.

But with just a little mental preparation, you will be able to navigate the seas, no matter how uncomfortable they may make you at first. If you know, for example, that you might get a headache from the lack of caffeine, instead of resenting the headache you can nod to it when it comes and just say, "Okay, this is going to be a tough few hours, but just for today, I can get through these feelings and stick to my program. This is temporary; I can do it. And it shows me how addicted my body has become to a powerful substance."

You might also feel a bit cranky, so if you can put off making important phone calls or having a critical meeting on a weighty issue, do so. Because you are not taking in artificial stimulants, you might feel a bit sluggish and uninspired to exercise. The last thing you may want to do is exercise, but do it anyway; within five to ten minutes, you will be glad you're on your bike, hiking, or on the treadmill. Exercise creates a natural sense of wellness by increasing blood flow and by creating endorphins that make you happy; your body can use the boost as you withdraw from the artificial stimulants. And with exercise you never have the crash that comes after a sugar or caffeine high. Drink lots of clean, fresh water and herbal tea. And add the following meditation to your daily routine.

If meditation is new to you, don't be shy. For many people the word brings to mind an image of sitting in an uncomfortably stiff position and feeling antsy or preoccupied. It is nothing more than the practice of quiet contemplation. You just turn your focus inward for a few minutes so you can access a deeper reality. But what a powerful few minutes they can be.

By practicing a daily ritual of closing your eyes and turning your thoughts to the shift or change that is being awakened in you, you can greatly accelerate the cleanse's positive effects.

Today's Meditation

Find a quiet spot and sit or lie down and close your eyes. For at least ten breaths, drop down as deep into yourself as you can and connect to the part of you that wants to heal and flourish. Feel the little buzz of magic that is getting stirred within, and repeat the following phrase a few times: *I am leaning in.*

By repeating these affirming words, you are gently but firmly planting the idea that you are beginning a process that will reward you in all dimensions—improving your health, restoring emotional connectedness, and making you more comfortable and confident about your overall sense of place in the universe. As you breathe into the words *I am leaning in*, feel yourself moving in the direction of realizing your highest and most fulfilling path. No pressure, no specific goals. Just a little push to help you gain momentum. Set your sights on how you would like to feel and do your best as you move in that direction. Imagine what a cleaner and more vibrant way of living will feel like.

As you say the words, know that you will naturally draw into your awareness whatever you need to understand or embrace. That's the beauty of meditation: you will receive inspiration. Don't worry about how long you sit . . . even a few breaths is a good place to start.

Now plot out what you'd like to eat tomorrow. Choose a couple of recipes from the back of this book or from a favorite cookbook, or think about what you can order from the cafeteria at work, and get excited about what the future holds. This is an ever-unfolding process of wellness, and there is much to discover. You might even ask a friend to share a meal with you so that you have some companionship as you learn about new things.

DAY 2:

Why No Caffeine?

THE FIRST THING MANY PEOPLE MISS IS THEIR MORNING COFFEE, especially in the first few days of the cleanse. Even those with impeccable diets and wholesome lifestyles often hold on to their beloved coffee. We love the smell, the taste, the whole ritual of waking up to it each morning, and of course we love coffee's mind-clearing effect. Going off it can be challenging. And caffeine isn't just in coffee—it's in black and green tea, many sodas, dark chocolate, and those ubiquitous energy drinks, too. It's also found in many over-the-counter medications for colds and headaches, like Excedrin and Anacin, because it enhances their ability to work quickly.

There's much about caffeine that taxes the body, and I find that focusing on its negative effects can help you steel yourself for going off it for these weeks. Just remember, I'm not asking you to give it up forever, though after going off it you might find that you want to try. There *is* life after caffeine, and it feels so good.

When we stop drinking coffee or other caffeinated beverages, within the first day withdrawal often sets in. The most common feelings are irritability, drowsiness, fatigue, headache, and anxiety. The side effects of withdrawal are short-lived, don't happen at all for many, and are fairly mild in most people who experience them at all. Nonetheless, caffeine withdrawal is considered serious enough that caffeine addiction was proposed as a substance-abuse problem to the American Psychiatric Association. The duration of withdrawal is estimated at a relatively short two to nine days for most people. By the end of the first week of the cleanse, you should certainly be over the hump.

What is it, exactly, that caffeine does to cause such havoc in our bodies? Caffeine is a central-nervous-system stimulant, which earns it the distinction of being classified as a psychoactive drug. It affects our perception, our mood, and our behavior. One of the things caffeine does is raise levels of the neurotransmitter dopamine in the brain, which temporarily increases feelings of pleasure. However, a dependency can build up very quickly and it takes more and more caffeine to get the same feeling of well-being.

Along with a dopamine increase, your central nervous system mistakes caffeine for adenosine, a naturally occurring chemical in your body that's linked to calming and sleep. What happens is that caffeine binds itself to adenosine receptors in the brain, blocking their effects. In the short term, you feel more alert (because the adenosine is blocked), but without the actual adenosine in contact with its receptors, levels of anxiety and restlessness can go up, and the *need* for sleep or rest remains. By ingesting caffeine you miss the benefits of rest and low anxiety that you would have had were the adenosine able to dock correctly.

Over time you also need more and more caffeine to get the same energy boost. This is how we end up needing three cups of coffee in the morning just to get going, and even more throughout the day to keep going. Of course, if you are this dependent on caffeine, you've also been experiencing energy crashes during the day and an overall feeling of exhaustion that can drain the spirit out of life.

Caffeine further exhausts the body by stimulating our adrenal glands to produce adrenaline. Adrenaline is part of the "fight-or-flight response," a biological reaction to stress. During this response, your body also produces higher levels of the hormone cortisol—the "stress hormone." Cortisol is considered a stress hormone not because it is inherently bad for you; in fact, in normal levels it helps with glucose metabolism, regulating blood pressure, lowering inflammation, and raising immunity. Cortisol also has some short-term benefits when it enters the bloodstream in higher amounts: it creates better memory function, enables a quick burst of energy, and lowers our sensitivity to pain.

In an ideal world, once the crisis is over our bodies can return to a resting state. However, modern life, and substances like caffeine, can all too easily keep our cortisol levels artificially high.

Some of the problems associated with stress fatigue and consistently high levels of cortisol, which overuse of caffeine contributes to, are lowered thyroid function, cognitive problems, decreased bone density and muscle tissue, higher blood pressure, lowered immunity, and an overall inflammatory reaction in the body.

It is interesting that the very things we take caffeine for—to get more energy and mental focus—are sacrificed over the long term by ingesting it.

In sum, caffeine keeps us awake longer than we should be and makes our bodies burn the candle at both ends to do it; in that way, caffeine could be considered a substance whose primary purpose is fooling our bodies into going against their own best interest.

With each day that passes, the effects of caffeine, and of withdrawal, will lessen, and your body can relearn how to go about its processes the way that it was designed to. Your brain will be able to work correctly and give you a natural calming effect, and your blood pressure won't have abnormal spikes. Your energy level will return to normal (and normal should be "high" if you are doing all the other things in this book) without the need to boost it.

A cup of coffee or tea here or there can be enough to stave off withdrawal symptoms and keeps the addiction limping along, so you have to cut it out entirely to discover its full effects on your system.

To completely avoid caffeine, you will also want to avoid foods that are coffee flavored, such as ice cream and yogurt. As far as chocolate goes, dark chocolate has the most caffeine. Even a small serving of dark chocolate can have up to 30 milligrams of caffeine in it, nearly the same amount as a can of cola (as compared with 90–150 milligrams in a cup of coffee and 30–70 milligrams in a cup of caffeinated tea).

These foods are verboten during the cleanse anyway, but now you have even more reason to steer clear!

And here's a word on energy drinks: the average energy drink on the market contains about 80 milligrams of caffeine in an 8-ounce serving. But many of them are packaged in 16-ounce cans, some even bigger; energy drink companies come up with larger sizes all the time so that they can advertise the massive doses of caffeine that they contain. In reality, most of them contain generally about the same amount of caffeine as a cup of coffee *per serving*, but one can often contains multiple servings.

An energy drink is merely a soda containing large amounts of caffeine as well as sugar, high-fructose corn syrup, or aspartame, if it's the sugar-free or diet variety. So, along with the caffeine, your body has to deal with a variety of other harmful substances. Drinking energy drinks will definitely give you a "buzz," but will tax your body even more than regular coffee or tea. Recent studies have shown that energy drinks actually raise the risk of stroke even in young men by thickening the blood, in a process that is not completely understood.

These drinks are basically just strong coffee with some other dangerous and untested substances. There are good things in some energy drinks—like ginseng—with known positive effects, but mixed with high levels of sugars and inorganic compounds, they are not a good bet for overall health.

Question of the Day: If I can't drink coffee, I may just give up on the cleanse altogether; I can't take the withdrawal . . . what should I do?

Okay, it's time for a compromise! I would much rather you lean out of the caffeine addiction gradually than give up the whole exercise of cleansing. I know that for a small minority of people, it can be just too rough to suffer the headaches and irritability, especially if you have a job that requires that you be "on" all the time. And I know how sluggish you might be feeling, but trust me, this will pass—especially if you're taking my advice to substitute ten to thirty minutes of exercise for your morning cup(s) of coffee. Here's a solution: wean yourself off coffee. Begin by cutting your regular coffee with decaffeinated coffee. You can create a mix of two-thirds coffee to one-third decaf for the first week. For week two, drop your coffee down to one-third real coffee to two-thirds decaf. And by week three, see if you can go without the coffee altogether. (Note: herbal tea is best, but decaf is fine until you get to the point where you can move to tea.)

Drink more water, and get lots of rest. Without coffee, you are likely to sleep better, and if you're exercising to replace your coffee, that will also help you sleep. You might want to sleep an extra hour at night or take a short nap during the day. Your body will recover soon enough, and you will feel energetic and clear.

What to Avoid:

- **Coffee, tea, caffeinated soda (or sodas with guarana), green tea**
- **Energy drinks**
- **Dark chocolate**
- **Coffee-flavored desserts**

- Over-the-counter medications containing caffeine (read those labels!)

Enjoy:

- Herbal tea
- Decaf coffee

DAY 3:

Lay the Groundwork for a Breakthrough: Meditation and Visualization

I THOUGHT I'D TAKE TODAY TO TALK ABOUT A COUPLE OF PAR-ticularly powerful tools for creating change in your life—and making change stick. I'm talking about meditation and visualization. Both these practices are invaluable to me, especially when I am pushing myself into new territory. They help me calm inner turmoil and ground and fortify myself to take on new challenges. Throughout the book you will come across some simple meditation routines. Today I want to look closely at what meditation can do.

A Few Facts About Meditation

Meditation is good for you physically, emotionally, and spiritually. By making a regular practice of it, you can expect:

- improvement in concentration and artistic abilities
- improvement in performance levels in sports

- increased ability to learn and communicate
- profound relaxation
- a change in metabolism due to the lowering of biochemical by-products of stress
- lowered heart rate and blood pressure
- greater ease of respiration
- a feeling of being "in tune" with your higher nature
- greater insight and inspiration
- a more grounded approach and response to life's challenges

Helpful Tip

To lean in to the practice of meditation, we'll start with a mini-meditation.

Try it now. Read through these instructions a few times and then simply put down the book and close your eyes. Count out ten breaths, focusing on the inhalations and exhalations. You can use your fingers to count down, so that you don't get sidetracked by wondering how many more breaths you have to go.

Try repeating an affirmation: *I break through,* for instance. Say "I" on the inhale, and "break through" on the exhale. By saying it, you will keep reminding yourself of where you want your energy to flow.

Ten breaths will take up slightly less than a minute, so you can't possibly have the excuse that you don't have time. You can do this practically anywhere (except while driving!)—on a subway, while drying off after a shower, or sitting in a doctor's office. The best time, though, is to sit with your eyes closed in the morning before you get going with your day. This way, the rest of the day will be seeded for calm, centered, and inspired focus.

As you become more comfortable with being still and present, increase the period of time that you sit; move it up to five minutes, then ten, and finally twenty. The amount of good you get out of it is truly worth the time spent.

Visualization

While meditation is more about being quiet and letting go so that you can receive insight and inspiration, visualization is a more active process of mapping out the changes you'd like to make in your life. When we visualize what we want to see happen in our lives, we give our brain new images and feelings to hold on to, thus providing both our mental and physical energy a new framework to fit into.

I liken this process to what happens when you add new track to a toy train set: until you lay new track (fresh images and new potential) and pull the switch so the train can transfer over (upgraded thought system), the train (your thoughts) is stuck going around and around on the same track (negative or self-defeating images). The old tracks will still be there, but you have expanded your options, given yourself some new routes to travel.

As you learn to switch up the images of yourself, everything else follows. You start gravitating more toward experiences and practices that support the new images. And really, that's how a quantum leap happens. You start looking at yourself and life with a new eye, a new perspective, and things just start feeling different. When you rejigger the way you perceive, you show up in your life differently.

When I began to visualize myself as being successful, for instance, I would see myself in my mind's eye as someone who was industrious and well connected and confident. Those visuals replaced the old ideas I had of myself as being timid and passive, unable to attain anything great or important. Regular practice reshaped and replaced the images I had of myself so that I began to know what it felt like to be someone who is successful. I played out in an inner arena what I would look and feel like, how I would proceed through my day, and the manner in which I would present myself.

After a few weeks of visualizing myself as successful, I was able to bring that fresh image of myself into my everyday life by making phone calls I had been afraid to make, and following through with ideas and projects, because that's what a successful person would do. And it wasn't a big challenge or struggle, because I had experienced it all in my mind first. Because I had done test runs in my mind, had already stepped into bigger shoes, when I took it out into the world, it already felt natural. I was in my new skin, and it felt right.

What we project out into the world starts with how we experience ourselves on the inside. Think of it this way: if you visualize yourself as healthy, slim, and energetic, you will most probably begin to hold yourself in a stronger and more poised posture. And then you will act in ways that a healthy, slim, and energetic person would act. You will undoubtedly eat better, exercise more willingly, and stick to your commitments so that the image of yourself is supported and substantiated. And then people will see and treat you as that strong and secure person, which will further energize your new way of being.

Visualization is a process that simply makes use of the fact that changes that are practiced in the mind first manifest much more readily on the material plane. It's just a matter of giving yourself new cues—new images and information—so that your behavior can follow suit.

Exercise

With this exercise we are going to work on a deep and energetic level. We are going to work on creating change in your inner life, so that you begin to show up in the world in a new way. We will be creating a shift in your core energy so it actually resonates with and draws to you situations, people, and opportunities that will help usher in a greater level of health and happiness. This is not magic; we can't simply want or imagine something and then expect that it will become so. Instead, you will be clarifying your intention, pulling in spiritual support, and training yourself to be the person who can sustain the transformation you want to experience. Simply read through the following passages, pausing to focus on the cues I give you. Or better yet, have a friend read it aloud to you so that you can completely move into a meditative state. You might also want to record your own voice and play it back so that you can follow along more seamlessly. (I have meditation CDs available on my website, www.kathyfreston.com.) Here we go!

Relax and get comfortable. Close your eyes and let yourself be carried by your breath into stillness, into your creative center. Let the chatter of your mind fade away, and put your focus on your breathing. Feel the air as it enters your nose and travels down through your chest and into your belly. Feel your belly as it rises and then gently falls, exhaling. As you enter into this work, engage all of your body, mind, and soul. Feel the weight of your body as it touches the ground beneath you; experience the solidity of your bones, the fluid motion of your blood and organs, and the immense complexity of all the different functions that are taking place within you physically. Notice your mind as you dip in and out of thoughts and images, time and space; simply observe it all, stepping back and into stillness.

And engage your soul, the part of you that is beyond your personality and history, beyond the external details of your life. Let your soul guide you into a more mystical realm. Begin to sense a veil being lifted with each time you inhale and exhale. You are becoming more grounded and centered even as you feel lighter and more expansive.

Now call in Spirit in whatever way feels right to you. You can imagine angels surrounding you, or guides, or you might just imagine a beautiful golden light that is pure love, pure benevolence. Feel the beauty and potential for miracles as you allow yourself to be washed through with all things good and light and lovely. Notice how this light that is all around you sparks to life the light that is already within you. Feel it as it opens your heart, releases your tensions, and lifts you to a higher vibration.

With your attention on this mystical presence, silently articulate your desire to have a breakthrough. Let it be known that you would like to experience a change or shift. Ask for an intervention at the highest level, that your desire comes to pass in a way that is gentle, yet powerful. And now clarify your reasons why you want this breakthrough to happen. Notice if you flinch at any of the reasons, and allow yourself to be completely honest about your agenda. Being truthful and integral strengthens the momentum of creation. Now tweak your desire so that it is oriented beyond simply your own self-interest, encompassing also the well-being and uplifting of the whole. Plant your seeds in a way that is not demanding or needy, but rather in a way that promotes and extends the love that is within you. Let it be known that you are ready to have things unfold, beginning right now, in the best way that would serve everyone involved.

And now, let's clear the way. Before any great passage, there are often obstacles and difficulties to overcome. This is our soul's opportunity to heal and expand. At this part of the meditation, you can address your fear and any trepidation that stands in the way of a successful breakthrough. It is important to hear the shadow voices within you, because if you try to suppress them or make them go away, they will just try harder to stand their ground and block your movement forward.

When you give permission to the wounded parts of yourself to speak, you actually make it possible for them to finally know peace and let go of their stranglehold over your psyche. This part of you only wants to process, receive compassion, and be accepted. Say to those voices of fear or doubt, "Okay, go ahead. Say what you want to say. I'm listening." You may see a flash of the child version of yourself as you let this part of yourself become known. Although you might not want to hear this voice or experience this communication, it is essential. When we allow for our shadow, we tap into the part of us that is raw and vulnerable and powerful. Making peace with all the different parts of ourselves liberates us from old and unconscious patterns of behavior. The more clarity and awareness we have, the more freely we can move toward our higher nature.

When you sense that your inner shadow has had its say, tell it, "Thank you. I heard you. And I appreciate what you've been through." And then, with the help of the spiritual presence you've called in, flood this part of yourself with love and light. Feel yourself being healed, cleansed, and loved. Completely loved and accepted. Feel the relief at letting go.

Now, in your mind's eye, allow a picture to come to life of your being happy, feeling free of worry, and experiencing the breakthrough you wanted. Hear yourself thrilling with laughter at the succession of good news and positive feedback. See everyone around you being supportive and joyful. Feel the quiet peace that seems to have encircled your world. Watch how your life changes subtly and gently, and at times even radically. Notice that it feels as if this was always meant to happen. Look around your inner vision, and see who is in the picture and who is not. Take note of your posture, your new demeanor, and how your energy has shifted. Notice how well you connect with people and how you seem to be coming from a much wiser and more empowered place. Feel the kindness of your heart as it radiates out. Celebrate the force of light with which you are getting comfortable.

Enjoy the success and let yourself ride the wave of this glorious breakthrough. Notice what you have had to let go of in order to achieve this new state of being, what changes you might have had to make. See flashes of healing as you realize what was holding you back. You need not control the images, just let them come. Feel this new energy settle into every cell of your being; let yourself be filled with the magic you always knew was on its way. Add as much color, intensity, and sound to your visualization as you can. And when you feel a click, as if it has gone as far as it needs to, let it go. Release your vision out into the ether.

It's time to say thank you. Stating your gratitude takes you into a "quantum"—or immediate—manifest place. Wanting something means you put your energy into hoping something pans out in the future. On the other hand, saying thank you for it (in advance of your actually seeing it manifest) injects a powerful energy into that seed of potential. Say, "Thank you for this breakthrough. Thank you for having this miracle unfold so perfectly, so beyond anything I could have ever imagined. Thank you for the ease and spirit of grace within which everything came together." Let the feeling of gratitude permeate your consciousness.

And now let it go. You have just completed some profound and committed work. You can release the details and timing to Spirit. Things rarely happen as we expect them to, so drop any need to control and oversee this unfolding miracle. Audibly sigh, releasing any leftover tension or expectations. Feel in your bones that you are on course and that the more you align yourself with the light within and all around you, the more easily, gently, and swiftly things will come to pass. Rest assured, your gift—in its perfect form—is on the way. And so it is!

This should take anywhere from ten to twenty minutes. After you do it once and you have a good feel for it, you can flash on the images briefly throughout the day, so that your new senses are continuously supported and bolstered. Even a quick image of yourself being the person you want to be is enough to shift your behaviors and patterns. Keep returning to the feeling you had during the exercise, and know that you are retraining yourself to be aware, strong, happy, and healthy.

DAY 4:

The Big Picture

YOU'VE MADE IT THROUGH THREE DAYS! THREE DAYS OF LETTING your body relax and stabilize. Three days of following through on your intention to get healthy. With every day going forward, you will feel better about your course—not just because you are taking good care of your body, but also because you are answering a deep-seated (and sometimes unconscious) desire to heal. Something inside you knows that this is right, and you will feel directed by an internal compass that urges you onward.

Consider that perhaps it was the dismissal of this inner compass that brought on gnawing and ambiguous guilt feelings over the years. I don't know about you, but I spent years crucifying myself every morning for whatever I'd done wrong the day before. Mostly, I didn't even know what specific crimes I had done to myself (body or spirit), but I knew I wasn't caring for things in the way that I should. I simply felt "off course." It's so nice to have a break from that feeling of being ill at ease. Knowing that you've been eating healthfully and without adding a toxic load to your already-burdened system is its own high. And with this cleanse, we are not only detoxing from years of putting junk into our bodies, but we are also letting go of old habits, beliefs, and ways of being that no longer serve us.

With this process, we are changing a few eating habits, but we are also working on aligning our behaviors with our spirituality, or sense of values. During these twenty-one days, I encourage you to keep your eyes—and your heart— open and to think deeply about everything that goes into feeding ourselves the diet we've become accustomed to. In this way you will become a conscious eater.

A part of the cleanse process is about considering the whole picture: how the food serves our body, how it affects the environment, and the process by which it gets to our plate. It means that we scrutinize the methods of production from beginning to end, making sure that what we eat is not only good for us, but also good for every-one involved.

We are shifting the way we eat from blindly answering our cravings or mechanically counting protein and carbo-hydrates to considering how our choices will land in every respect. By thinking more deeply about the food we eat, we begin to see beyond our own personal self-interest and toward the good of the whole. In this way, we not only heal ourselves, but we become the healers this world so sorely needs.

Helpful Tip

Before sitting down to eat, ask yourself:

> *How can I eat in a way that is kind, responsible, and attuned to the needs of my body?*
> *What can I do to bring my life to the highest vibration possible?*

You may not have all the answers yet, but by simply asking the questions you will set in motion a process of ever-increasing consciousness. Just slow down enough to ponder the big picture, and soon enough, it will begin to come into focus.

As you go about this, please be sure to enjoy some delicious foods like brown rice, quinoa, steamed or sautéed vegetables, chickpeas, yams, rice cakes or flax crackers with almond butter, apples, blueberries, hot whole-grain cereal with chopped nuts and fruit with soy milk poured over it . . . Remember to take pleasure in the food that is abundantly available to us!

Today's Meditation

I open my eyes so that I might heal. What a powerful statement. It means I am ready to confront the darkness within (the parts of myself that care only about immediate or personal satisfaction) and the darkness in our world. By nudging myself to open my eyes, I will begin to see what needs to shift on a fundamental level. By healing myself and becoming more aware and thoughtful about my choices, I am also offering that light and healing outward into the world.

DAY 5:

Move Your Body

FOR A PART OF THIS CLEANSE, YOU ARE WORKING ON YOUR IN-ner life by confronting the old systems of thought and be-havior that hold you back. You are clearing away old traditions and passed-down beliefs that no longer serve you. And you are simultaneously working on yourself in tangi-ble—external—ways: cleaning up your diet, meditating, vi-sualizing, and approaching relationships in an elevated manner. You also want to be sure you are bringing your body up to speed in terms of strength and flexibility, so that you are as strong in body as you are now becoming in mind and spirit! Today we'll focus on ensuring you a good workout for the duration of the cleanse—and beyond.

How Much?

A good workout four to six days a week is ideal. If you don't already have a program, start by doing something every other day, and then move toward exercising more steadily throughout the week. If you can get your heart pumping for at least twenty or thirty minutes at a stretch (to the point where you're breathing hard but can still carry on a conversation), you are doing really well. Hiking, brisk walking, jogging, dancing, boxing, and riding a bike on an incline are all perfect ways to get a cardiovascular workout, which makes your heart and lungs stronger and more capable of handling life's stresses and strains. Playing competitive sports like tennis and basketball are also great to get you sweating and stretching.

It's important to work some strength training into your program—push-ups, weights, or challenging yoga, for instance. By building muscles, you keep your bones strong, because when you lift heavy weights (or the weight of your own body), you force your bones to adapt to the exertion placed on them by producing matrix proteins, which fortify them. This is a highly effective way of preventing osteoporosis, a weakening of the bones.

By undertaking a program of strength training for at least a few days a week, your muscles, tendons, and ligaments become stronger, making your body better able to protect itself from the stresses that cause injury. And of course weight training also increases your metabolism, because as your muscles get bigger, your body uses up more calories even while resting.

Exercises like tai chi, yoga, or chi gong require you to use your focus to maintain balance and concentration while increasing coordination, which sharpens your responsiveness and ability to think clearly. It is said that a supple spine is the key to youth and vitality because "life force" can move freely and easily through a flexible spine. You might think of how a tree weathers a windy storm; it bends without breaking.

Make a Plan

Because it's all too easy to get swept up in your day without leaving yourself time to work out, it's best to budget in a little time for exercise. Right now, look at your schedule and find an hour or so to hit the gym or trail at least four days a week. If it's written into your day, you will find a way to schedule other things around it. This time is for you; it's not a luxury, it's a necessity for your immediate and long-term health. When four days a week becomes comfortable, bump it up to five, and then six. Let your increasingly beautiful body inspire you to become ever more athletic and committed to your program.

Helpful Tip

Upon rising in the morning, sit at the edge of your bed and stretch. Take a deep breath and get your blood and oxygen circulating. Stand up and reach for the ceiling, and then swing your arms in a few circles, backward and then forward. Then bend from your waist and touch your toes (or try to!), letting your muscles awaken to the day. Bend side to side, and roll your shoulders back so your chest is open and you feel strong.

Whenever you can think about it throughout the day, stretch. By extending your body and keeping it open, you will be reminding yourself to stay supple while you push yourself to new levels of strength. If you have a few minutes between calls or errands, drop to the floor and do ten push-ups. And then the next chance you get, do fifty sit-ups. Or even ten. You'll be surprised at how all these little efforts add up. Instead of making a gossipy phone call, or surfing the Net, you can give your energy a little jolt by doing something constructive.

Did You Know?

Exercise is good and necessary for the body to thrive, but it is also beneficial for our emotional well-being. When you get a good workout, you feel good about yourself for making the effort, and you certainly feel good when people look at your physique admiringly. That's the obvious stuff. What may not be immediately apparent is that anxiety and depression are eased by exercise, because when you move your body and get your heart rate going, endorphins are produced, which bring on a feeling of well-being.

In a recent study at Duke University, exercise was found to be more effective in beating depression than Zoloft, the often-prescribed antidepressant and anti-anxiety medication. Although Zoloft worked more quickly to alleviate the troublesome symptoms, after ten months of steady exercise (walking briskly on the treadmill a few times a week), the test group in the research experiment was significantly less depressed than the medicated group. Exercise gets the brain to produce serotonin, dopamine, and noradrenaline—all the same neurotransmitters that are targeted by the pharmaceuticals—and it may do a better job of regulating them. These naturally occurring neurotransmitters are raised by intense strength training or prolonged aerobic exercise, and each contributes to feelings of energy, clarity, and alertness. Of course this is not to say that people should not use psychotropic medications when all else fails, but it is certainly worth giving a good and consistent workout a try, since it carries no ill side effects at all! (Note: Never go off any medication without a doctor's supervision.)

According to Dr. Dean Ornish, research shows that exercise "may even help you grow . . . new brain cells," which would affect memory and cognition, making you feel more on top of your game.

Lastly, Dr. Woodson Merrell, author of *The Source: Unleash Your Natural Energy, Power Up Your Health, and Feel 10 Years Younger*, says that "nothing raises your energy faster and more effectively than exercise. The simple act of moving can jump-start your metabolic machinery. . . . Oxygen utilization becomes more efficient; sugar is processed better; fat and calories burn faster; brain cells regenerate quicker; you think more clearly; your heart gets bigger and stronger; the balance of your nervous system shifts toward the calming aspect (parasympathetic); and your emotional happy switch gets turned on by the release of neurotransmitters." He explains that because our genome is the same as our hunter-gatherer ancestors', whose lives consisted of roaming around and finding food, we are designed to move. So when we move, we kick into our natural energetic programming.

Overall, exercise increases the muscle-to-fat ratio, which makes you leaner and stronger. It enhances your everyday tasks and makes you feel good about yourself. And best of all, when you work out, the body produces "happy" chemicals, neurochemicals that make you feel good and at peace.

Today's Meditation

Today, *I move.* I breathe deeply, open my body, and get strong. I cherish this gift of flesh and bones and muscle that gives a home to my soul, and I celebrate this body of mine by moving in ways that bring me to new levels of vitality. I see this task as joyful, and as much as it may be difficult to push myself, I love knowing that I am on the move in a positive direction. I move, I open, I strengthen.

Day 6:

A Break from Alcohol

For five days now you've stayed away from alcohol. Today we'll look at why it's on my Big Five list. Of course, if you don't drink at all, giving it up is a nonissue. If you drink to excess or are struggling with an addiction, please keep an open mind about how you might address this. It's well beyond the scope of this book to address alcohol addiction; if you suspect you may have alcoholic tendencies, I suggest you check out Alcoholics Anonymous (AA) online. The questionnaire you will find there will help you to determine whether or not you have an issue with drinking that needs attention. I also write about addictions fairly extensively in *Quantum Wellness: A Practical and Spiritual Guide to Health and Happiness*, and you might want to start there.

There are many studies out now that suggest that we derive some health benefits from moderate drinking—to the heart, the nerves, to easing self-consciousness. I certainly won't argue against that. Most people do enjoy social drinking. Tensions ease, the stressful day recedes into the past, and you can just enjoy the moment. Not only is drinking alcohol a festive activity to be shared among friends, but it is also a form of self-medicating from the basic stress of existence. This is why humans have used it for so long and in so many cultures. But alcohol has some less than healthy effects on us, even in moderate amounts, and that's why we abstain from it for the duration of the cleanse.

Alcohol can impair our judgment and slow down our cognitive responses. In slightly higher amounts it can supercharge our emotions and land us in situations we'd never have tolerated sober (fights with friends, getting in a car with someone who has also been drinking, etc.). Drinking alcohol can also lead us down a fairly slippery slope, where that glass or two of wine a few times a week becomes a glass or two every day without our noticing, and pretty soon that amount isn't quite giving us the effect we're looking for, so we pour a third glass and then a fourth. There are biochemical reasons for this, and to understand how it happens, let's look at how alcohol works in the brain. The discussion will get a little technical. Just bear with me.

How Alcohol Works in the Brain

Alcohol can interfere with the brain's chemical messengers, specifically the neurotransmitters serotonin, GABA (gamma-aminobutyric acid), and dopamine. Neurotransmitters will either encourage and quicken, or slow down and cease, impulses between neurons in the brain, dramatically affecting our moods, our ability to think clearly, and the signals the brain sends to the body. It's not a stretch to say that how our neurotransmitters are functioning affects how we experience the world and ourselves.

Serotonin affects our thinking patterns, memory, appetite, body temperature, and endocrine regulation. Dopamine is involved with feelings of pleasure and reward. (That's why it is affected by nearly all addictive drugs. Stop feeding your brain these pleasure-giving substances and dopamine levels go into instant decline, making you acutely aware of its absence, which is why it's so hard to quit.) GABA is involved in memory and cognitive functioning. Alcohol ingestion has, to a greater or lesser extent, some impact on all these functions. How does that happen?

For one, drinking alcohol temporarily increases the level of serotonin in the brain, which in turn increases its influence on mood and thinking, elevating each. This is why we often crave a drink at the end of a tough day. Stress and modern life decrease our serotonin level, and alcohol is one of the quickest and easiest ways to raise it. Once you take a drink, that alcohol begins circulating throughout your bloodstream within five minutes. Your serotonin level goes up and you feel better.

However, this is just an artificial boost, and those serotonin levels can fall just as fast as they rise. On top of that, excess alcohol, or continued use, can actually lower serotonin levels overall, causing mood swings, depression, and other problems related to serotonin depletion. It also interferes with the essential amino acid tryptophan, the precursor to serotonin; tryptophan has been called "nature's Prozac," and although that is an overstatement, it does help us feel relaxed, with a general sense of well-being.

GABA, by contrast, is an inhibitor, meaning it inhibits

signals between neurons, and alcohol heightens its effect. Since GABA is involved in many areas of the brain, multiple functions will show signs of slowdown. The most obvious are motor skills. Sluggish motor response can be seen in anyone who has "had a few." This can also affect memory, making associations and connections slow and difficult.

As for dopamine, which is associated with reinforcement behavior and feelings of reward, alcohol boosts its level as well. These increases can easily lead to the loss of inhibition and judgment, a quality that makes alcohol consumption so popular! Dopamine also gives one a feeling of well-being, and when it is in decline, the urge to raise it again can be overpowering. After the initial effects of alcohol wear off, dopamine levels fall below their normal nondrinking state. This is another reason why even moderate drinkers can feel deprived if they don't have a glass or two.

Alcohol has strong effects—not all of which are understood—on these neurotransmitters, each of which has some effect on one or more of the others. But what *is* clear is that drinking even moderately does not leave us with our nature-given brain chemistry, and that we do drink, in large part, to affect that chemistry. And even beyond that, our brain chemistry is actually affecting our desire to drink. See the vicious cycle we can get caught up in?

Let's take a deeper look at the mechanism through which alcohol is metabolized in the body: metabolism is the process by which the substances we eat and drink are converted into other compounds, most less toxic than the original, some more. Because our bodies treat alcohol as a toxin, a poison to be purged (because, for your liver, that's exactly what it is), it is detoxified and removed from the blood through the process of oxidation. The liver is where most of the metabolism takes place.

But the liver can only metabolize a certain amount of alcohol in any given time, no matter how much is consumed, and that rate is affected by genetics, which vary from person to person. Generally, the liver metabolizes alcohol more slowly than the body absorbs it into the bloodstream, so when we drink, a certain amount of the alcohol nearly always affects the body and the brain.

Curiously, alcohol does not raise your blood sugar level. In and of itself it will actually lower it. What does raise our blood sugar level when we drink are the carbohydrates contained in the drink, and that is what is turned into glucose in our body. Alcohol actually inhibits the liver from releasing glycogen (carbohydrates stored in the liver and released for energy when you're between meals), which is how it lowers blood sugar overall. Your liver treats the alcohol like a toxin and goes about the detoxification process, putting off releasing glycogen until it is complete. And since this is a slow process, that means you can go without a steady release of glycogen for a long time, which can lead to hypoglycemia (low blood sugar).

Further compounding their effects, most alcoholic drinks have a high simple carbohydrate content because of the sugars in them (i.e., the grapes in wine, the malt in beer or Scotch), and this will flood your system with glucose. Your pancreas releases insulin in order to handle the glucose at the same time that the liver is impaired by detoxification. What you can get is a fluctuating blood sugar level, with all its attendant problems (including insulin resistance). Something to keep in mind: good health depends on stable blood sugar levels.

This is why it is much easier to give up sugar and alcohol at the same time. If you were to try to quit one without the other, you'd still have to deal with destabilized blood sugar levels and the quitting would be much harder. You might notice a friend who has given up drinking alcohol addictively turn to eating sweets in large amounts; this is because their system is used to being loaded up on sugar, and they haven't quite gotten off that old sugar/insulin roller coaster. To achieve a healthy state of equilibrium, it's wise to forgo all the substances that will throw your system back into the old craving cycles.

Alcohol causes stress-related issues in the body as well. One way is by raising cortisol levels. Cortisol is the "stress hormone," and elevated levels of it can destabilize blood sugar levels and also add fat to the body by keeping us in a continuous, low-grade fight-or-flight metabolism. Alcohol also depletes vitamins B_6 and B_{12} as well as folic acid—nutrients the body needs to cope with stress—and can interfere with REM sleep, leaving you less rested when you wake up in the morning.

The Benefits of Taking a Break

So, you see, alcohol puts stress on your body in a number of ways and an occasional break does your body a favor. You give your brain a chance to find its natural, uninterfered-with chemical balance. Your body is once again able to produce serotonin at healthy levels, and this includes recovering from its daily depletion from stress without artificial stimulation. You are able to keep dopamine in balance so your brain isn't always craving a drink to temporarily elevate its levels. The fact is, if given the chance, the brain has an amazing capacity to readjust neurotransmitter levels and effectiveness all by itself, and clearing it of alcohol frees it to do that.

Also, by reducing the toxin load, you give your liver the opportunity to regenerate itself (unless it has already experienced serious scarring—cirrhosis—from heavy drinking). And the liver is brilliant at doing this. Remember, your body reacts to alcohol as though it were a poison and the liver gives priority to metabolizing it out of the system, putting on hold the important function of releasing glycogen to stabilize blood sugar levels. If you want your liver to heal itself from a lifetime of heavy (or even mostly moderate) alcohol use, and you want to see your blood sugar levels reach the optimum range for good health, it is a good idea to give yourself this kind of "vacation."

For me, however, the biggest reason to abstain from alcohol for the length of the cleanse is to break out of habitual behavior and just see what's going on. It's usually perfectly healthy for a woman to have three or four drinks a week (for men, two to three drinks a few times a week is usually fine), but I know that if I'm not careful, I can find myself having a couple of drinks a night simply because I'm not paying attention. It's good to step back in a meaningful way every now and then and see how I do socially without "numbing out" or "loosening up" with a drink.

It's important to know that we don't have to rely on alcohol to deal with stress or have fun. And if you steer clear of alcohol for even twenty-one days, your body will have the chance to reset and find its balance, and that's always a good thing.

Just Notice

If you are used to drinking a little wine or other alcohol, take note of how your body feels the morning after an evening without wine or spirits. You are probably more clearheaded than usual, and without that gnawing feeling of, "Oh, I think I drank a little too much yesterday." You don't have to have a hangover to know that you've overindulged, for alcoholic drinks act a lot like sugar—a quick high, and a sluggish low soon to follow. Your body has to produce a lot of insulin to counter the effects of the drinks as they break down into sugar, and that means you feel overwrought and fatigued. And studies have shown that although an occasional glass of wine won't show up on your waistline, it can affect your risk of getting cancer. Dr. Neal Barnard, president of the Physicians Committee for Responsible Medicine, says that women who have even one glass of wine or other alcohol each day— if it's every day—have a slightly higher risk of breast cancer, compared with women who drink only occasionally. The problem is that alcohol disrupts folic acid, a B-vitamin that is involved in our anticancer defenses.

You've been avoiding wine, beer, and spirits. Here's what you *can* enjoy:

- Sparkling water with a twist of lemon or lime or a smidge of unsweetened pomegranate juice
- Any kind of chilled herbal tea served in a festive glass
- Good, old-fashioned water

The Lean

As important as it is to go off alcohol during the cleanse, I don't want you to end up not enjoying your own birthday or the festivities at a wedding. Have a drink and enjoy yourself if your cleanse overlaps with a special occasion. Perhaps cut that glass of white wine with some sparkling water instead of drinking it full strength, or have only one glass of champagne to toast the good news rather than drinking throughout the evening. Also, if you slip up, just do the best you can moving forward. Just because you don't do everything perfectly on the cleanse doesn't mean you should give it up altogether.

DAY 7:

Rest

AND ON THE SEVENTH DAY . . . WE'RE GOING TO FOCUS ON SLOW-
ing down and allowing yourself to rest.

Before I committed to the path of wellness, I used to be
in the habit of pushing myself beyond the point of exhaustion. It's so easy to fall into that trap, as you probably know.
It is achievers who do self-work—and if you bought this
book, you're in that category of people who take the time to
test and improve themselves—good for you. For all of us,
there is always so much to do and not enough hours in the
day to do it (as my mother always said). But this is not the
time to follow the credo "Don't stop till you drop." In fact,
now is the time to begin to understand the value of balanc-
ing work with rest, relaxation, and sleep so that your body
can reach a healthy equilibrium.

I know, I know. I can just hear you writhing. "Well,
that would be nice, but I have kids and deadlines and bills
and. . . ." But nothing! Rest is critical to your health. And happiness. Yes, you have to live your life with all its regular de-

mands, but you also have to give yourself the time and space to heal. Do what you have to do to keep your life running, but make a point to take some time to rest during the cleanse.

Sleep and Rest

You need seven or eight solid hours of sleep in a dark room (if there is light leaking in, it will alter the production of melatonin, a naturally occurring hormone that regulates diverse body functions and has antioxidant properties). This allows the body to get to the deep work of repairing what is tired, rebuilding what is worn out, and fighting potential disease or infection. Have you ever noticed how you can go to bed feeling ill, but after a good night's sleep wake up feeling healed? Research shows that this might be because, while we're asleep, levels of certain immune-system proteins rise, but drop again when we are awake. If you are feeling unwell, rather than jump to the conclusion that you need medicine, take a warm salt bath to relax your body and have some hot herbal tea, and then climb into bed. The body is wise and industrious; if you give it half a chance, it can often heal itself.

Sleep, the Almighty Healer

Keep the following in mind in case you are tempted to insist on a rigorous schedule, especially now, when you should be more quiet and calm than usual.

- **Nothing can revitalize the nervous system like regular and nightly deep sleep. If we don't** give ourselves that time, our nervous system won't recharge and will thus be unable to send the correct impulses to our organs for optimum functioning.

- It is during the time of decreased activity that the body can do the deeper, and often neglected job, of detoxification, repair, and rebalancing.

- When we sleep deeply, the body produces HGH (human growth hormone), which encourages the restoration and maintenance of bones, tissue, and muscles. This happens much faster and more efficiently than during waking hours.

- We are more resistant to infection when we get proper sleep, while those who are sleep-deprived see a reduced level of white blood cells—an essential part of the body's defense system.

- When we get regular sleep, our body's circadian rhythm ensures that our hormones are properly regulated. Adrenaline and corticosteroids drop, and we therefore feel more relaxed and balanced. And testosterone and fertility hormones are secreted, helping us to feel strong and vital (and sexual).

- Our metabolic rate increases during deep sleep, so even as we are resting, we lean toward a healthier and slimmer body!

All these processes occur during "regular" life, but it is even more essential during the cleanse that we give our body the gift of sleep so that it can get to the more arduous task of deep detoxification and rebalancing. Rest is the great rejuvenator, so invest in your health by giving your body what it needs.

Speaking of Rest

To better understand how rest and relaxation are critical to healing and overall health, I consulted the work-life expert Joe Robinson, and this is what he had to say:

> Rest and recharging are essential for enabling the mind and the body to replenish resources. After a long day, week, or year, we're no different than an iPod or cell phone that's run out of juice. You wouldn't expect your iPod to spontaneously recharge itself after it has run down. Same for humans. We need to get charged up again. I call it the Refueling Principle. Stepping back to relax and unwind brings our brains and bodies back to life. We're in the knowledge economy, so it's how fresh your brain is that determines whether you thrive or not. MRI scans of fatigued brains look exactly like ones that are sound asleep.

> Time spent off-task is medicine. An annual vacation has been shown to cut the risk of heart attack in men by 30 percent and in women who take two vacations a year by 50 percent. Where else can you get a benefit like that? What we learn from the science is that the time itself

helps the healing process. Vacations can cure burnout, the last stage of chronic stress, which is very difficult to get rid of. But it takes two weeks for that recuperative process to occur. So the time is key to regathering crashed emotional resources, such as a sense of social support and mastery. Research shows that your state of mind, like the physical body's condition, is all about conservation of resources. If resources get depleted and are not replaced, we get sick. If you're regularly replenishing mental, emotional and physical resources through refueling, rest, and recreational activities, you're insuring that you can thrive through the toughest demands. It's like a bank, and if you overdraw your resources, you're spent.

Leisure time and relaxation are huge stress buffers. If you don't make time for rest and play because you're too caught up in the false urgency of busyness, the stress never gets relieved, so it spirals and becomes chronic, leading to a host of issues, including digestion problems such as irritable bowel syndrome. The hormones released by the fight-or-flight response set off by stress, such as cortisol and adrenaline, reduce immune function. Stress also plays havoc with your thinking, letting the emotional center, the amygdala, hijack rational thought and ratchet up impatience, irritability, and anger, which undermine health. Another interesting thing that happens when you're run by hurry-worry and nonstop busyness is that you lose the ability to control impulses. You have to check your BlackBerry every two minutes. You have to grab another Twix. You have to have another nightcap. Stopping lets us step back and return command to the higher brain, remember where we're going and why we're going there. We get back in touch with who we are and our priorities.

The bottom line is that no matter how important your work is or how pressed you are for time and energy, you will not ultimately thrive in achieving your goals if you don't let go and relax every once in a while. If you burn out, you won't be any good to anyone and you certainly won't be enjoying a significant upsurge in your health or sense of well-being.

Helpful Tip

Take a few minutes to sit in the sunshine—or in a beautiful spot out in nature—and soak in the beauty. Look around and see how life thrives without our pushing it to do so. The trees grow and flowers bloom; day turns to night, the seasons change, and the complex ecology thrives on its own. Notice how life has a cycle of pushing forward and resting, of action followed by stillness.

During this time of cleansing and renewal, curl up in a blanket and read a book with a cup of hot tea, or watch a movie with your partner or best friend on the weekend. Play some meditation music as you catnap for twenty minutes in the middle of the day, and let the gentle sounds carry you into a restful state.

If you find yourself getting worried about what you "should be doing," grab some paper and make a list of the things you need to do. Remind yourself that you can get to them later in the day or in the next few days when you are feeling recharged. Then do your best to let them go. This is your time. Delegate as many tasks as you can so that the regular busyness of life doesn't cut into your sanctuary.

Go to bed early with a good book, and sleep in as much as you can during these twenty-one days.

Today's Meditation

As much as this process is about being proactive and changing our habits, it is also about allowing the body to do what it innately knows how to do: process and let go of the old; heal; and rejuvenate. So today, I say to myself: *I trust the intelligence of my body.*

Week Two

Day 8:

Traveling, Eating Out, and Other Challenges

As you are probably discovering, it's a good idea to do the cleanse with as much stability in your schedule as possible, knowing you have a pantry full of options that you can turn to when it's time to eat. When you are in control of the menu, you are much more likely to stay within the cleanse guidelines *and* eat a variety of foods you like. But of course, most of us live busy lives—with work obligations and dinner invitations—and these often challenge our resolve to stick to the plan. But with just a little preparation, you'll be able to travel and dine out without stumbling.

Question of the Day

How do I remain on track when I am traveling or if I go to someone's house for a dinner party?

When I travel, I always bring along a few things that I know will get me through a tough spot if I can't find any healthy food. For instance, I always have a Ziploc full of almonds or mixed nuts to snack on while waiting in an airport or between meetings. Nuts are high in protein and unsaturated, heart-healthy fat, which can help you to feel full longer so that you eat less when you actually sit down to a proper meal. In addition to satisfying a hunger pang, by choosing nuts to snack on you are feeding your body some good nutrition.

Women in a Harvard School of Public Health study who ate five or more 1-ounce servings of nuts per week actually saw a 30 percent reduction of risk for type 2 diabetes compared with those who did not eat nuts regularly. Besides the protein, nuts also deliver healthy doses of magnesium, fiber, and zinc.

You can eat them straight out of the bag or sprinkle them into some soy yogurt or over a breakfast of hot cereal. You can mix them up with some dried goji berries for an extra dose of antioxidants, or even blend them into a smoothie to add texture. Nuts really are miracle foods packed with nutrients, and although they have about 225 calories per quarter cup, the science indicates that they are slimming—perhaps because they're packed with fiber, perhaps because they fill you up quickly and inhibit your desire to eat other foods. Especially while you're on the cleanse, you should carry some nuts with you for those times when you're hungry, so that you have no reason to "cheat."

When you're going to be out and about, try to carry a couple of pieces of fruit with you. Apples and pears are my favorite choices. Both are high in vitamins C and A, calcium, and dietary fiber. Granny Smith apples are the absolute best choice because they are the lowest of all apples in sugar content, but any kind of apple is fine. And remember, no matter where you are, you can pretty much always dash into a supermarket and purchase some (preferably organic) fruit and nuts to hold you over for a while.

In addition, I suggest you stay well stocked with energy bars so that you can grab one as you're running out the door. I like the ones that are vegan (dairy free) and sweetened with stevia, brown rice syrup, or agave nectar. My favorite brands also include freeze-dried greens in the ingredients, so that I can enjoy getting another dose of vegetables when I snack or have a meal replacement. Another thing to carry is a nice little selection of herbal teas, as sometimes we just need the comfort of something warm and soothing. These days you can often find soy milk or creamer just about anywhere to make it even more of a treat.

When staying at a hotel, I like to start off with oatmeal for breakfast. I always ask that they make it with water instead of milk or cream, and have found most hotel kitchens to be accommodating. With some fresh blueberries on top and a little steamed soy milk if they have it, it's a substantial way to begin the day. If it's hot outside and I feel like having something light, I usually opt for a fruit salad. Later, for lunch or dinner, I order a hearty soup (lentil, minestrone, tomato) from the room-service menu and ask if they can prepare something using every vegetable they have in the kitchen. With a baked potato drizzled with olive oil or a big salad on the side, I will have covered all the necessary nutritional bases.

If I don't feel like I've gotten enough protein (although that is usually not a problem, what with nuts or bean soup or

protein bars on hand) I will shake up a packet of protein powder, which I carry for a quick fix, in a bottle of water. Choose
a brand that says "vegan" on the package; there are many delicious ones that contain soy, rice, or pea protein. You can mix
it up with water alone, or ask the hotel kitchen to send you
up a blended fruit smoothie with soy milk, and just fold in
your protein powder. I wouldn't make a habit of this latter version, though, as it might be a bit too much fruit and sweetened
soy milk (hotels often don't have unsweetened soy milk).

If you're headed to someone else's house for a meal (or a
weekend), just call ahead to let your host know that you are
on a cleanse and won't necessarily be sharing in all the
meal(s). If you feel awkward doing this, just be sure to explain
that you don't want anyone to go to any trouble at all and that
you're looking forward to their company. If the situation is
right, you can offer to bring along a dish or two. That way
you'll be sure to have food on your plate and you won't risk
sitting there looking like a party pooper. Ever since I've han-
dled it this way, with the advance call and all, no one has
had an issue with my "strange" eating habits, and, in fact,
my experiment usually turns into an interesting conversation piece.

A Little Story

I remember one time when I didn't call ahead to the host of
a dinner party, and things got pretty uncomfortable.

It was a few years ago. I was doing this cleanse and my
husband and I were invited to another couple's house for dinner. We didn't know them well, but I looked forward to spending some time with them in the intimate setting of their home

with about twelve other dinner guests. Not two minutes into the evening I had to decline the offer of a cocktail (reminding myself that this was not forever, just three weeks), which was hard to do since I was a little nervous. Instead I sipped on some sparkling water and tried to laugh along with everyone as they went into the party zone.

When dinner was served, I passed over the chicken entrée and said, "Oh, thank you, but I'm just in the mood for the vegetables, if you don't mind. And the rice pilaf looks wonderful, too!" The host shot me a rather annoyed look. I felt a wave of mixed emotion, but what was I supposed to do, have the chicken just to please her? She didn't say anything and neither did I.

But when she got around to serving dessert—a divine-looking chocolate cake—and I opted for some of the fresh organic berries I had brought as a gift, our host laid right into me in front of everyone: "Darling, you are *such a bore*. For all our sakes, loosen up!"

I felt like shrinking into the size of the pea on my plate. I was so embarrassed and didn't know what to say. I knew I was not being the ideal guest, but I was handling it in the best way that I knew how. I didn't want to have a drink just to make her feel better; I didn't want to eat meat just to fit in. I didn't want to get my blood sugar and insulin back to the mess it had been before just to be polite. But still, I really wanted to be accepted and liked!

An Added Lesson

As I sat there trying to figure out what to do next, I realized that this experience was testing more than the depth of my commitment. In fact, it was bringing me face-to-face with one of my oldest social issues—the intense desire to be liked and accepted. Growing up nerdy and unpopular had had its way with my self-worth! I saw just how much I needed to witness this insecurity so that I could finally deal with it; I needed to face that old desire to be part of the "in" crowd and realize that there were values more important to me than fitting in. I was maturing, and that maturity was being cultivated in the awkwardness of *not* going along with the plan.

By opting to stick to the guidelines of the cleanse, I chose being healthy and conscientious about my body and the foods I chose to eat over a few moments of social acceptance. Yes, it cost me a bit of humiliation, but I came out feeling that I had chosen well by not compromising what I knew to be right. I tried my best to be gracious and not call attention to myself, but the rest was not in my control, and I had to accept that people would not always be pleased or in agreement with my choices. The bottom line, I realized that night, is this: as long as I am not dogmatic or judgmental of others, I will have done the best I can by staying true to myself.

Of course, I'm not being fair to my host here: she had no idea what I was doing, so it's not entirely fair of me to frame it this way. I should have told her, and since I've taken that very easy step ever since, I haven't had this sort of embarrassing experience again. So the episode was a doubly important learning opportunity for me, and I apologized to my host afterward for not having explained my situation.

Our challenge as humans is always to love the part of ourselves that is rejected and disowned. When we come to terms with the part of us that is vulnerable, we arrive at a deep inner peace, and thus are able to act in the world a bit more peacefully. That was one profound lesson from that awkward dinner party.

The way is not always easy or comfortable when we want to upgrade or break out of an old mold. *And* we have to do it anyway. We need to be resourceful as we go along through our day, and we need to continue educating ourselves on how to be healthier and more conscious. But we need to do it in a way that makes room for other people to grow in a manner and at a rate that is comfortable to them. It's interesting isn't it, how this process of cleaning out not only detoxes the body, but also detoxes the psyche?

This much is for sure: healing is multidimensional. It isn't just a matter of getting the physical stuff on track or training ourselves to be thoughtful consumers; it's also about reaching back to old emotional wounds and letting life teach us with the experiences that come to pass. When we approach the cleanse and everything about our personal development from this perspective, the momentum of healing rolls with a greater thrust.

Today's Meditation

Throughout the day today, I will remind myself: *I am flexible*. As I repeat the words, I feel myself being able to roll with whatever comes my way. I may have to make do with some quick fixes for food when I am pressed for time. But there are new foods I am growing to love, and new friends who share my values and interests.

As I practice saying *I am flexible*, and resist the temptation to grab onto old ways or to defend old fears, I am beginning to sense life carrying me to a wholly new stage of unfolding. I get stronger as I am challenged and figure things out; I grow more assured of who I am, and navigating my new path becomes easier every day.

DAY 9:

Meet Your Shadow

BY TODAY, YOU MAY BE FEELING A LITTLE ANTSY, THOUGH YOU are probably past the withdrawal stage, if you even had one, for everything you've given up. The first few days usually have their own kind of excitement as you dive into a process that promises to transform you in so many ways. That awareness alone creates a momentum. And anyway, we can all go a few days without the things we're used to. But by today you may have started missing your old rituals and habits. You might have had a bad day at work and just want to relax with a martini. Perhaps a friend ordered a juicy cheeseburger at dinner last night, and you wanted to join him in his carnivorous and carby bliss. I understand. By Day 9, it can sometimes start to feel like "Enough already. I'm not so sure about this."

These thoughts and feelings used to come up for me, too. Instead of fighting and resisting them, I decided just to observe what was going on inside me. Instead of caving to the impulse or, on the other end of the spectrum, beating myself up for not being strong enough to succeed, I would just try to think, "Wow. This is interesting. What is this resistance all about?" I'd sit back and observe the chatter in my head.

What became clear to me was that I didn't like giving up my attachments. I resented not being able to turn to those little pleasures that I had grown so used to and even dependent on. Half a pot of coffee made creamy and sweet to gear me up for the day. A thick turkey sandwich and chips for lunch with a tall soda. A piece of cake or some cookies at around 4 PM. Some version of a meat-and-potatoes dinner accompanied by a glass (okay, a couple of glasses) of wine. Margaritas on the weekend always accompanied by cheese and crackers. These were the traditions of my days—actually, they were the traditions of my parents, too, and partaking of them was in my bones. But as time and years went by, I had come to realize that these traditions were not serving my health at all. The half pot of coffee did not always do the trick to wake me up, and I had begun to feel an acidic stomach after even one cup. The sandwich was hearty, but I was eating so much bad fat and processed carbs and not getting that much nutrition, and I'd feel really heavy after eating. Same with dinner. I also noticed, with a bit of concern, that if wine was not available, I would get annoyed. And trying to change any of these things always sort of failed: *I liked them. I didn't want to give them up.* Not even for only twenty-one days.

But then I thought: Should that desire, that habitual urge to just feed myself what I wanted, override everything? My health? The way I look and feel? Is my attachment to these gustatory pleasures so strong that I choose them over my health and personal evolution? The answer, of course, was no. I had to challenge myself. And if that meant I had to process some anger or frustration or resentment along the way, so be it.

I know it's not easy. Of course it's not. We're talking about breaking patterns and habits that you've been "perfecting" for years! If these feelings are coming up for you, try this next exercise. It may feel a little goofy at first, but I'm guessing it will become a tool you use often, not just on the cleanse but whenever you're facing something particularly challenging.

Exercise

For those of you who are not used to introspection, this exercise is probably going to be difficult, and you may feel very awkward. But please do it. I'll bet that once you do, you'll be so glad you did that you may even find it becoming part of your regular coping process.

First, get out a journal and write down every single thing you feel anxious or angry about. Whether or not your complaint is rational doesn't matter; your feelings exist and they need to be tended to so that they don't fester and create havoc in your life (or persuade you to go off the cleanse).

Now place two chairs so that they face each other, and sit down in one of them. At this point, please make sure you have privacy so that no one walks by and thinks you're ranting!

As you face the opposite chair, conjure up a version of yourself that is the "raw" part of you; put this image out in front of you and make it as real as possible (even though it's really more a sort of energetic projection). You may think of this presence sitting across from you as your soul, wise guide, inner child, or simply the purest version of yourself. With your journal in hand to remind you in case you forget something, begin to speak out loud—rail even—about everything and anything that is bothering you. Twist up your face and use your body as you express how furious you are at feeling unsatisfied and unhappy. Yell! Scream! Cry! Say all the things you dared not say before. Give (loud and expressive) voice to the feelings that have been lingering just beneath the surface, perhaps kept down by some addictive eating or drinking habits. Now is the time to let it all hang out.

When you feel like you've reached a natural lull, or you have said all that you can for the moment, get up and move to the other chair. Now you are embodying that highest version of yourself. Some people find that it helps to pretend that they are talking to their best friend, who has just unburdened her- or himself. If you're like many overachievers, you are merciless with yourself, but forgiving of others. If you act like it's someone else, rather than you, who is angry and frustrated, you'll probably be kind and forgiving—because that's the kind of person you are. Well, give yourself a break, too.

Hold your hand over your heart and gently say to the angry and frustrated you who is sitting across from you, "I hear you. I understand." And then just let whatever wants to be said come out. Remember, you are now giving voice to your deeper, wise self; if a punitive or judgmental voice comes out, you are not yet connected with this inner light. Give it some time until a compassionate and kind voice makes itself heard.

When this part of you has had its say—it has imparted

some advice or wisdom or simply let you know that you are loved and accepted—move to the other chair and say, "Thank you. I'm sorry I haven't checked in with you for a while. But I'm here now, and I will do my best to keep showing up." If you feel there is more to say or work out in this session, continue in the same vein until you feel a click of completion. Throughout the day, or whenever you feel out of sorts, check in with this part of you that is forgiving, compassionate, and wise.

We all have things to process throughout the day, and throughout our lives. If we want to break the addiction cycle—to negative feelings, or food, or whatever it is that has us thinking we can't be free from it—we have to face the very things that anger or scare or repulse us. Once we turn toward the so-called demon with mindfulness, the demon softens. And in that little measure, we are healed.

Ask yourself: When I am not assuaging my discomfort with any of the Big Five, what feelings begin to come up? Am I willing to deal with them? A "negative" feeling is something like a bully; it tries to get your attention in an annoying or bothersome way. If you don't heed the little fella, he comes back swinging harder. He wants you to pay him some respect! The good news about bullies, though, is that they often melt in the face of compassionate attention. They don't know what to do with themselves. So as you go along these next few weeks (and, really, for the rest of your life) ask yourself throughout the day what you are really feeling. And then just sit with whatever comes up and apply some compassion. Process all that you need to in order to get things moving, and then feel yourself being filled with light and comfort and love. Be assured that grace is in this exercise and that your wellness evolution is the ultimate goal.

Today's Meditation

Throughout the day, I will say to myself with eyes closed, *I examine myself.* I will always be challenged by various situations—relationship conflicts, stress at work, drama with my kids—and thus experience feelings that are uncomfortable. All of this provides the friction necessary for my personal growth. If everything went along swimmingly all the time, I would never have the opportunity to stretch myself, or work at pushing through the obstacles that keep me stagnant. In order to keep moving forward, I can step back from the feelings and examine them, noting how familiar or repetitive they are. I can think about how and when they originated so that I understand the historical progression. By realizing that we are all wounded in some way, I can look to my wounds as an opportunity to know myself better. As I come to know myself better, I will find myself connecting with other people on a deeper and more meaningful level. As I now see it, the purpose of my life is to grow and awaken to the powerful potential that is within. My most sacred mission is to focus on moving through the places that hold me back.

Day 10:

Cooling Digestive Fires: Gluten and Your Gut

TODAY WE'RE GOING TO LOOK AT ANOTHER ONE OF THE BIG Five, gluten—both what it is and how it affects our health. I find that many people don't know that gluten can be a source of health problems. The fact is, many people don't tolerate gluten well, and they have no idea what it's been doing to their system until they give it up. It is often the root cause of ongoing digestive complaints, from general gassiness and bloating to irritable bowel syndrome and celiac disease. Cutting it from the diet can largely reverse these problems. This is not to say that gluten isn't perfectly fine for a lot of people (it is for me), but it's a good idea to cut it out for the twenty-one days so that you can gauge whether or not you are adversely affected.

What is gluten, exactly? It is the key component in most types of bread, and it's found in a number of grains—namely wheat, rye, and barley. It is part protein, part starch or carbohydrate, and is the substance in flour that helps with rising and gives baked goods a fluffy texture. However, although we generally think of gluten as being only in bread and pasta, in fact it is now widely used in processed foods, with negative consequences to many people's overall health. It's important to check labels and read ingredients carefully. Other names for gluten include: modified food starch (though this sometimes refers to corn), hydrolyzed vegetable protein, hydrolyzed wheat protein, textured vegetable protein, and, of course, wheat. The more highly processed a food is, the more likely it is that these ingredients will show up.

Gluten is often present in:

- Bagels
- Beer
- Bread & bread rolls
- Cake
- Cookies
- Couscous
- Crackers
- Deli meats (which are heavily processed)
- Flour, including wheat, spelt, semolina, and rye
- Muffins
- Noodles
- Pancakes
- Pasta
- Pizza
- Sauces (often thickened with flour)

There are gluten-free versions of these products available made from beans, rice, corn, nuts, soy, and potatoes. These are the foods you'll want to choose during the cleanse.

Did You Know?

It seems that gluten was discovered by seventh-century Buddhist monks who were looking for an alternative to meat for their vegetarian diet. Gluten is made of wheat flour and water: the dough is soaked in cold water to remove the starch. The remains are a gummy mass primarily made up of gluten, which has a unique texture that makes it capable of being molded into an edible food with the consistency and appearance of meat.

Gluten is often used as a substitute for meat because its appearance can be almost disturbingly similar to meat, giving people the feeling that they are enjoying old favorites (chicken patties, duck, ground beef) without the animal protein. And it is high in protein. Gluten is added to many processed foods because it is so adaptable and can easily substitute for more costly ingredients, like meat. When manufacturers realized they could save a lot of money by adding gluten to their products, its use became ubiquitous.

As an additive, gluten can be found in practically any processed food. Not only is it used to stabilize, thicken, and add flavor, gluten also gives structure and texture to mass-produced foods that would otherwise not be very appetizing. When you eat a bagel or a pizza, the chewy texture is most likely achieved through the use of gluten. It is commonly added during processing because it's a way to instantly increase the amount of protein in an otherwise protein-deficient product.

Along with gluten, it is common for manufacturers to use other harmful food additives, such as monosodium glutamate, or MSG (which does not actually contain gluten, despite the similar-sounding name), sugar, salt, and hydrogenated fats. In almost every case, along with chemical additives, the very nutrients that were leached out of the whole food in the manufacturing process are also added back into the final product. These products are (ironically) then labeled "enriched." A fact that's missing from processed-food labels is that every time a food is processed into another form, the energy you get from it is less and less potent. When you eat whole foods, your body does the processing, and your body reaps all the benefits.

What Happens When You Eat Gluten?

Gluten is not a naturally occurring protein in the human body. In fact, some researchers call gluten protein a toxin. How could something that we eat so much of be classified as a toxin? Some studies suggest that gluten damages the small intestine and allows food proteins to be released into the body, and the immune system then interprets these proteins as invasive and goes into high gear to defend itself. In other words, you get an overblown immune response. This kind of immune response can possibly contribute to or mimic diseases like lupus, arthritis, and multiple sclerosis.

So, in affected people, gluten causes general inflammation of the intestinal tract and can also damage the small, hair-like projections in the lining of the small intestine, called villi, which are involved in the absorption of nutrients. Although inflammation starts off as a good thing—when we are cut or have an infection, the body creates swelling to seal off the injured area so that the repair work on the damaged tissue or bacteria can begin in a protected space—it can also be a double-edged sword with an excessive and out-of-control inflammatory response, spreading out and attacking healthy tissue. This out-of-control immune response and inflammation is what researchers say is the beginning of many disease processes, cell proliferation and malignant (cancer) transformation included. Anytime you can avoid creating inflammation in your body, do. It's best to keep equilibrium.

Now on to digestion, which is the engine of our health. Problems that take place in the digestive system can cause an array of health issues. Problems with digesting gluten exist along a spectrum. At the least harmful end of the spectrum, gluten in the diet is suspected to cause headaches, asthma, skin rashes and hives, weight gain and/or loss, bloating, fatigue, and behavioral problems such as depression. At the most harmful end of the spectrum is celiac disease. Commonly thought of as an allergy, it is actually an immune-system response to gluten. Initially, research suggested that celiac disease was relatively rare, but with more awareness and more research, scientists are realizing that celiac disease is not rare at all—about one in 133 people have it, and many of those people will have no symptoms at all, meaning every day they are damaging their bodies without knowing it. This number doesn't include the people who are diagnosed with gluten sensitivity, which is thought to be even higher. Many people who are sensitive to gluten's effects will never know it, but will suffer for their entire lives from various preventable health problems.

The good news, though, is that usually the damage is not permanent. The small intestine is capable of healing itself through a strictly gluten-free diet. Once a person with gluten sensitivity or celiac disease starts a gluten-free diet, the positive health results are immediate and dramatic.

If You Have Kids, You Might Want to Know

Recent studies have shown that gluten might contribute to autism. In fact, there are parent groups that take autistic children off all gluten products (along with dairy) for a period of at least three months because of the remarkable success rate of those children who maintain a gluten-free diet. Children who made the dietary switch began making eye contact with their parents for the first time and attending regular classes at school rather than special ed.

Because undigested gluten has the ability to attach itself to the opiate receptors of the brain (as does casein, a protein found in milk), the opiate effect can become addictive, behaving like a powerful, mood altering, brain-damaging drug. Perhaps that's one of the reasons why we can feel "addicted" to bread, bagels, cereal, and the like.

As you aim to eliminate gluten over the course of the cleanse, your best bet is to avoid most processed foods, unless they are labeled "gluten-free." Gluten-free foods are becoming more and more widespread in grocery stores as awareness of the problems that gluten can cause becomes better known. Nearly any health food store now has a wide selection of products that are identical to "normal" foods— just without the gluten. The benefits of a gluten-free diet can be felt immediately, often within a few short days. For many people, the effects are so dramatic and so positive that the entire family goes gluten free. It is worth the trouble, because when the small intestine is able to heal and your body can actually process all the nutrients you eat, you will feel the difference and your overall health will improve substantially.

All this said, if you don't have any sort of gluten issue, the vegetarian wheat-gluten protein, called seitan, is a tasty, high-protein alternative to meat. (But don't eat it until after the cleanse is over!)

The Lean

For many people, gluten will be the hardest substance to avoid, because it is in so many things. There are tests available that can help determine if you are gluten sensitive, but they're not 100 percent accurate. That's why I have you cut out gluten completely while on the cleanse. Your best determinant is how you feel. Just be sure to add it back slowly when the cleanse is over. See how your body responds. You might indeed be fine with some seitan or a bagel (I am), but then again you might not. Let this cleanse reveal to you whether gluten is a wise food choice for you.

Please don't sweat the small stuff. Just do the best you can. This cleanse is not about achieving some sort of purity or perfection. Pay attention more to the larger amounts present in breads and pastries, rather than the trace amounts of gluten that might be in sauces or salad dressings. And as always, stick with food that is simple and unprocessed. That alone will keep you on track. Beans and whole grains, tofu and tempeh, vegetables and salads, fruits and nuts are always your best bet.

DAY 11:

Have a Little Fun

JUMP-STARTING YOUR PROCESS OF HAVING A HEALTHIER BODY, mind, and spirit can be hard work, but it should also be fun. Why? Because if we don't have fun, we lose out on the joie de vivre—the very joy of life that sustains us and inspires us to keep going! For many of us, it's hard to take the time just for "me"; we think there are always things we should be doing. We feel guilty giving ourselves some downtime, and continue to jam our schedules tightly with errands and obligations. When we neglect ourselves, though, we get run down. We burn out. Or get depressed.

So today I want you to spend as little time as possible thinking about the cleanse and have yourself some plain and simple fun. Don't analyze it too much, or worry that you are doing it correctly. Just dance to your favorite song, or play with your dog in the backyard, or get out some watercolors and paint something crazy. By taking fun seriously, we regain a quality of innocence. We shake out leftover tensions, and get our minds off the heavier subjects of life. I know that usually, when I put aside my worries or efforts to watch a funny movie or blast some good music, things have a way of working themselves out. When we hold too tightly to our goals, without stepping out and letting go, we lose our creativity. When we cut loose, new ideas just naturally flow into us. We feel refreshed, energized, and rejuvenated.

Exercise

Make a list of seven things that you love to do and that make you happy.

1.
2.
3.
4.
5.
6.
7.

Now slot one of those things into each of the seven days of the week. If you don't have a lot of time, just give yourself a quick blast of joyousness. For instance, when I'm getting ready for the day, I sometimes crank up my favorite songs and dance around the room as I make the bed or get dressed. It may not be the ideal fun session, but I sure do get a smile on my face that lasts me for a lot of the day. Rent a comedy and invite a friend to watch it with you. Roll around on the floor with your kids. Or put your dogs in the car, roll down the windows, drive up your favorite stretch of road, and just enjoy watching them soaking up the fresh air.

It's these simple things that often give us our most ecstatic moments. We feel lifted and carried by a sort of magic. And those moments bring in optimism; they remind us to love life. When we get silly, we feel the weight of our responsibilities slipping away, and we feel free. Those freedoms touch us at the deepest levels, and give us precious memories to look back on as we write the history of a life well spent.

Today's Meditation

I am happy, and I am free! I rejoice in my innocence and celebrate the gift of life. No matter what is going on, I can laugh. I can be silly. This levity makes my spirit soar. I am happy, right now, and I am free!

DAY 12:

The Trouble with Animal Protein

FOR MANY PEOPLE, ONE OF THE HARDER THINGS TO GIVE UP during the cleanse is meat. People do love their meat, be it a burger, chicken breast, or the occasional steak. If you're a carnivore, I applaud you for giving it all up for the duration of the cleanse. It's been almost two weeks, and my guess is you're already discovering how good it feels to eat just plant protein and whole grains and that you can be perfectly healthy without eating any animal products at all.

People on or off the cleanse decide to give up meat for a lot of different reasons: ethical, environmental, and personal health concerns among them. Today we're going to look at what animal protein does in the body and why it is not the healthiest choice.

Let's start by looking at what protein is.

Proteins are the building blocks of life. They are created through the linking of amino acids in various sequences and are part of every cell of your body. They perform many different functions, ranging from giving form and structure, aiding in digestion, and providing movement. Ligaments, muscles, hair, fingernails, organs, some hormones, even the lens of the eye are all made up of protein. Protein is also involved in getting oxygen to blood cells by making up part of hemoglobin. It is no overstatement that the human body cannot continue to live without protein.

Our bodies use a pool of about twenty amino acids to make up proteins for many different uses. We are able to produce fourteen of them ourselves and have to get the others from the foods we eat. Because our bodies are constantly constructing proteins at the cellular level and eliminating old ones, we need a continual supply of amino acids from food to keep the process balanced.

When we eat foods with protein, our bodies begin to digest those foods and break them back down into the component amino acids, and these in turn are used to produce various new proteins for the body.

According to the Harvard School of Public Health, animal and plant proteins are not different so much in their quality as in how the proteins are presented to the body and what other nutrients accompany them. A portion of meat may have a high density of various essential amino acids, but it also has loads of saturated fats. Proteins from legumes and grains, on the other hand, can deliver an equal number of amino acids with little saturated fat. Plant proteins also come in a package that contains a whole host of nutrients that are vital to our health: they're high in fiber (animal protein has no fiber) and high in the vitamins and minerals that our bodies need. Plant sources of protein also contain antioxidants, which are critical to neutralizing cancer-causing free radicals in the body. A varied plant-based diet, then, is a protective diet—sufficient in amino acids for protein needs; high in fiber, antioxidants, vitamins, and minerals; and low in saturated fats.

Specific animal products carry other health risks as well. Let's take a look at these.

Eggs

According to Dr. Michael Greger, director of public health and animal agriculture at the Humane Society of the United States, eggs are essentially cholesterol and salmonella delivery devices. We shouldn't be eating them at all. For starters, salmonella causes chronic arthritis and gastrointestinal disorders, especially in children. A hundred people every year come down with salmonella poisoning from alfalfa sprouts, so the Centers for Disease Control says no one should eat alfalfa sprouts—yet a *hundred thousand* are infected by eggs each year, and that doesn't produce the same indignation. Imagine if terrorists distributed bacteria-infested products across the nation and poisoned that many people. Yet people don't even blink when our egg industry does it every year.

Greger goes on to say that although cage-free, organic, and free-range eggs are better from a food-safety point of view, they have pretty much the same nutritional profile, and certainly the same amount of cholesterol. That means they also pose the same risk to our cardiovascular health. Salmonella may kill hundreds of Americans every year, but heart disease kills hundreds of thousands.

Eggs also have about ten times the hormone content of

meat and dairy, which means that prepubescent children are especially at risk.

There is protein in eggs, but you can get all the protein you need from plant foods like legumes, and all the "baggage" is good: legumes are loaded with fiber, folate, and phyto-nutrients, all wonderful things that aren't found in eggs and other animal products.

Dairy (Milk, Cheese, Butter, etc.)

Many of us grew up hearing that dairy is the best source of calcium. We still hear this all the time. The trouble is, it's not true. Despite all those clever "Got milk?" ads, milk and dairy products not only aren't the best source, they have been linked to higher rates of breast cancer and prostate cancer as well.

Dairy products do contain calcium, as well as some other nutrients, but along with that calcium comes a lot of unhealthy saturated fat and animal protein. You don't need to consume extra fat just to get the small amount of calcium that some dairy products contain. Dark, leafy green vegetables such as kale, chard, and collards are good sources of calcium and vitamin K and folate, and have little or none of the fat. The same is true for soy milk. And so-called "2 percent" milk may be 2 percent fat by volume, but it's about 33 percent by calories, which is what actually matters. I have to admit that I find this level of duplicity frustrating—shouldn't the government require that the dairy industry tell people that "2 percent" milk is actually one-third animal fat?

In addition to high levels of saturated fats, dairy products also contain casein, a protein that, according to Dr. T. Colin Campbell, author of *The China Study*, has been shown to promote cancer development. His work has been published extensively in the top scientific journals and was funded by the National Institutes of Health, a highly regarded organization that prides itself on its careful research. Dr. Campbell also reveals that casein and other milk proteins have been shown in sixty years of studies to "dramatically increase blood cholesterol and its associated lesion that leads to heart disease."

If you do a Google search for "dairy" and "Crohn's disease," you'll find extensive scientific evidence of a connection that deserves a lot more coverage in the media: Johne's disease in dairy cows, which is on the rise, is related to Crohn's disease in humans, which is similarly and probably not coincidentally also rising.

As Dr. Michael Greger explains in his lengthy analysis of the science on dairy consumption and Crohn's disease, which you can find easily online, "The best way to describe the disease to nonsufferers is to have them think of the worst stomach flu they ever had and then try to imagine living with that every day. Since the 1940s, there has been a rapid increase in the incidence of Crohn's disease in the U.S. and around the world, especially among people in their teens and early twenties."

Dr. Greger continues: "The U.S. has the highest rate of Crohn's ever recorded. The U.S. also has the worst epidemic of a similar disease among cattle, called Johne's disease, known to be caused by a bacteria called *Mycobacterium paratuberculosis* (MAP). There is now growing clinical, epi-demiological, immunological, experimental, and DNA evidence that this bacteria is the cause of Crohn's in people who drink milk from infected cows." I won't go on, but if you're still consuming dairy, you might want to further explore this possible link; please go online and read Dr. Greger's entire paper.

Fish

In recent years, many people have turned to fish because of the known dangers of red meat and chicken. Unfortunately, the news about environmental pollutants in fish just keeps getting worse and worse.

A lot has been written recently about mercury contamination from fish. Mercury is found naturally in the environment but recently has increased dramatically in volume, primarily from coal-fired power plants and various other forms of heavy manufacturing around the world. Coal-powered plants in China can affect the fish caught on the West Coast of America. Mercury has become nearly impossible to avoid in marine settings. The by-products of these industries have made their way deep into the food chain.

Mercury is found in especially high concentrations higher up in the marine food chain. It starts out by accumulating from the atmosphere into waterways, where it is changed by bacteria into methyl mercury and absorbed by small marine organisms. Small fish eat those organisms and accumulate mercury in their muscles (it binds to muscle proteins) and then larger fish eat them, acquiring dangerous levels that cannot be cooked out or purged before we eat them.

Methyl mercury is known to cause impaired neural development in unborn children, which is why the Environmental Protection Agency and the Food and Drug Administration were forced in 2004 to advise that pregnant women, nursing women, and small children limit their consumption of fish.

In adults, mercury is a neurotoxin, meaning it attacks the central nervous system. The effects of ingesting mercury are serious and numerous—fatigue, depression, memory loss, muscle and joint pain, and headaches are all believed to be among the "subtle" results of mercury in the diet.

Among the chemical by-products now present in the food chain are PCBs, or polychlorinated biphenyls. Before being banned in the late 1970s, these chemicals were used in many different industries, including manufacturing electrical parts and as an additive for paint and cement, among other uses. PCBs accumulate in the body over time. Fish can contain extremely high levels of PCBs. The harmful health effects of PCBs include impaired neurological development in children, and they are probably carcinogenic. They are hard on the liver as well. The liver detoxifies noxious compounds that our bodies come into contact with through breathing, eating, and drinking. PCBs can add greatly to that burden and should be minimized in our diets as much as possible.

The bottom line is, fish isn't a safe alternative to meat after all.

Chicken, Beef, Pork, etc.

What about chicken, beef, and pork? Perhaps you remember back in high school those little strips of litmus paper that tested a substance's pH. Just a little refresher: the pH scale is measured from 0 to 14, with the optimal pH balance in your body at a neutral 7. Your stomach has to produce a large amount of hydrochloric acid to digest meat—much higher, more concentrated quantities than it needs to digest plant-based foods—and this disrupts your natural pH balance, moving it toward acidity.

Generally, excess acidity can lead to inflammation and fatigue, and is associated with an increase in the risks of certain types of cancer, including pancreatic cancer, according to the *Journal of the National Cancer Institute*. Meat can also cause cancer because of the way its often overcooked. Meat contains a protein called creatine. When this protein is heated to very high temperatures, carcinogenic compounds are formed.

And then there is the weight issue. Obesity is close to being the most prevalent and preventable cause of death in the United States. The research of Dr. T. Colin Campbell has shown that diets higher in animal protein are correlated with higher rates of obesity.

At this time, nearly one-third of all American teenagers are overweight, and this problem almost always follows them into adulthood. What people seem to be unaware of is how easy it could be to shed enough weight to get to a healthy body size. The Western diet is incredibly high in protein; in fact, it's estimated that the average American eats at least *twice* the amount the FDA recommends, most of it animal protein (which the FDA doesn't recommend consuming at all). By simply making the choice not to eat animal protein, we could significantly cut the obesity rate and all the preventable health problems that come along with it.

Why are animal proteins associated with weight problems? Remember, most animal protein comes with a good amount of fat. The average chicken now has three times as much fat as it did just thirty-five years ago, so that even chicken without visible fat comes in at more than 20 percent fat, just as much cholesterol as beef, and zero complex carbs or fiber. As Dr. Barnard explains, a "20-percent-fat food with no fiber, no complex carbohydrates, and a fair load of cholesterol is not a healthy food, and that's what chicken is."

A diet rich in animal protein also puts us at greater risk of cardiovascular disease. That's because the high levels of saturated fat in animal foods take their toll on our hearts. The underlying cause of cardiovascular—or heart and blood vessel—disease is atherosclerosis, which is essentially constant damage to your arteries. This damage comes from elevated levels of low-density lipoprotein (LDL, or "bad" cholesterol), which itself comes from eating foods with extremely high levels of saturated fats.

Over time, LDL, whose normal function is to carry cholesterol from your liver to the rest of your body, instead provokes a response in your arteries, causing them to produce a substance that narrows them, making it difficult for blood to get through.

Your body does need some "good" cholesterol to maintain itself, but it manufactures all it needs—there is no dietary need to consume additional cholesterol, and the science indicates that consuming it is bad for us. A vegan (plant-based) diet helps you maintain good HDL levels and keeps LDL levels in check.

In a recent research study by the Physicians Committee for Responsible Medicine, people with type 2 diabetes who ate a low-fat vegan diet saw their indicators for heart disease dramatically lowered.

Again, eating meat has been linked with cancer. This seems to be, among other things, a problem of inflammation. Dr. Andrew Weil, who has popularized the field of integrative medicine, says that among the many problems with meat is something called arachidonic acid, or AA. AA is a pro-inflammatory fatty acid that is found only in animal products. Dr. Weil explains that "heart disease and Alzheimer's—among many other diseases—begin as inflammatory processes. The same hormonal imbalance that increases inflammation also increases cell proliferation and the risk of malignant transformation."

When you eat meat, and Dr. Weil points out that even chicken is full of arachidonic acid, you are stoking the fires of the disease process. It doesn't matter if the chicken is free-range or the beef is grass-fed. The offending fatty acid is natural and inherent in the meat.

Dr. T. Colin Campbell's research also indicates that a diet rich in animal protein is linked to higher rates of cancer. He says that "perhaps up to 80 to 90 percent of all cancers, cardiovascular diseases, and other forms of degenerative illness can be prevented, at least until very old age, simply by adopting a plant-based diet." This from a man who grew up on a dairy farm, got his Ph.D. in animal nutrition, and worked on a project to produce animal protein more efficiently.

Campbell found that, in addition to causing cancer, animal protein also fuels cancer that already exists. So you can have a carcinogen in your body, but it doesn't get "turned on" until you ingest animal flesh. Animal protein causes the carcinogen to become active and make mischief in the body.

And just a word on the efficacy and safety of the popular high animal protein diets, in case you are still tempted to believe that they are the way to lose weight: Dr. John McDougall calls high-protein diets "make yourself sick" diets, because they literally make you sick—the lack of carbohydrates sends your body into ketosis, which is basically starvation. So do they work for six months or a year? For people who can stay on them, they do. Of course, a crack or methamphetamine addiction, or chemotherapy, would also cause you to lose weight while making you sick and sending your body into shock. And like a drug addiction or chemo, a high protein diet is not something you can sustain, which is why 30 years after Atkins first proposed a high protein diet for weight loss, every dietary and medical body in the world has condemned the plan as unhealthy, and not a single study has supported it as something viable for long-term weight loss. Your body simply can't stay on the diet, and once you go off the diet, your body reacts as though you've just been starving (because you have) by making you even heavier than when you went on the diet in the first place. So you may lose weight more quickly, but the weight comes back and then some. And you have quite probably done your body harm.

The Immediate Health Benefits of Eating a Plant-Based—or Vegan—Diet

1. More energy. When you switch from eating a diet intense in animal protein to one that incorporates healthier, more varied sources of protein, you may immediately notice that you have higher energy levels. Why does that happen?

   Animal protein weighs your body down literally and figuratively. Your liver and kidneys have to work hard to digest and assimilate animal protein into a form that your body can use. When you stop eating animal protein, your body can use the vitamins, minerals, and antioxidants that are abundant in a plant-protein-based diet.

2. Clearer skin. Many people have also observed their skin clearing up when they switch to a vegan diet: animal meat contains animal hormones, and these hormones may exacerbate skin blemishes in some people.

3. Alleviation of chronic conditions, like arthritis. For many rheumatoid arthritis sufferers, dairy products are literally the cause of their pain. Eighty percent of milk protein comes from casein, and casein is believed to aggravate arthritis. People with the swollen joints and pain of arthritis have reported dramatic improvement when they eliminated all dairy products from their diet. Even skim and nonfat milk contain casein.

Some plants get their color from carotenoids, a plant pigment that you're sure to notice every time you go to the produce section of the grocery store—plants rich in carotenoids are usually yellow, gold, or orange. In 2005, researchers at the University of Manchester Medical School found that plants rich in certain carotenoids have antioxidant properties that lower the risk of rheumatoid arthritis. (Note: plants in the nightshade family, including tomatoes, potatoes, and eggplant, can exacerbate rheumatoid arthritis symptoms.)

To Sum It Up

I realize I have thrown a lot of information at you today, but with awareness comes resolve. The more aware you are of why it's so important to change the way you eat, the better you will be able to stick with the program. With this knowledge under your belt, the cleanse will feel less like a restriction and more like the upgrade that it is. And should you decide to maintain these upgrades after the completion of the cleanse, you will do so with the awareness that you have made a profound lifestyle choice with far-ranging, lifelong positive benefits.

DAY 13:

Questions for the Doctor

YOU'RE MORE THAN HALFWAY THERE. CAN YOU BELIEVE IT?

I've been doing the cleanse for so many years now, the twenty-one days are now almost as easy to get through as (fruit-juice-sweetened, wheat-free) pie. But I remember, when I first started, I had so many questions, particularly nutritional or medical ones. As I talk to people who are just now trying the cleanse or have only done it a few times, I realize that most of us worry or wonder about the same things. So for today, I've gathered together some of the most frequently asked questions sent in from readers, and I've asked Dr. Neal Barnard to weigh in with his medical expertise and insights.

1. How do I make sure to get enough iron if I'm not eating red meat?

The most healthful sources of iron are "greens and beans." That is, green leafy vegetables and anything from the bean group. These foods also bring you calcium and other important minerals.

Vegetables, beans, and other foods provide all the iron you need. In fact, studies show that vegetarians and vegans tend to get more iron than meat eaters. Vitamin C increases iron absorption. Dairy products *reduce* iron absorption significantly.

To go into a little more detail, there are actually two forms of iron. Plants have what is called nonheme iron, which is the ideal kind because it is more absorbable when the body is low in iron and less absorbable when the body already has enough iron. This allows the body to regulate its iron balance. Meats, on the other hand, have heme iron, which barges right into your bloodstream whether you need it or not. The problem is that many people have too much iron stored in their bodies. Excess iron can spark the production of free radicals that accelerate aging, increase the risk of heart disease, and cause other problems.

So while it is not good to be anemic, you also do not want to be iron overloaded. It is actually best to have your hemoglobin on the low end of normal. If your energy is good and your hemoglobin and hematocrit are at the low end of normal (a doctor can give you a blood test for these), that's a good place to be.

Having said that, you will want your doctor to review your laboratory results and track them over time. If your hemoglobin and hematocrit are dropping, that may be a sign of blood loss. That can be from benign causes, such as menstrual flow, but can also reflect more dangerous health issues, such as intestinal bleeding.

2. I notice that I'm feeling a little sluggish since I gave up caffeine. What can I do to bring back my regular energy?

Try a little extra exercise. Don't push yourself too hard until you feel like you are "over the hump." If you are new to exercise, try walking briskly in your neighborhood for twenty minutes, increasing the time and speed every few days. If you already have a good exercise routine, step it up as you feel comfortable. Add some extra weights to your resistance program, and try a more advanced yoga or Pilates class.

3. Is this cleanse safe for children and teenagers?

Vegetarian, especially vegan, diets are excellent for children. A diet of whole grains, beans, vegetables, and fruits is healthful for children, greatly reducing the risks of obesity, heart disease, cancer, and other problems later in life.

Planning is important for any sort of diet, of course. You'll want to be sure that children get adequate calcium, which is found in beans, greens, and many fortified foods. Also, it's essential that children take a multiple vitamin.

[You might want to check out an informative book on this subject called *Healthy Eating for Life for Children,* which was put out by the Physicians Committee for Responsible Medicine.—*KF*]

4. I am unable to eat soy because of an allergy; what can I eat on the cleanse instead?

You can focus more on eating lentils and legumes other than soy. You can also add in seitan—which is gluten—for protein. Remember, the guiding idea behind the cleanse is progress, not perfection! Unless you feel some digestive disturbance from the gluten, it's all right to compromise here. There is a grain called quinoa that is a complete protein. If you eat a variety of vegetables and some fruits, whole grains, beans and legumes, you will be fine. In some cases, allergies will change over time. For example, it is common for children to have allergies that disappear as they get older, and that occurs in adulthood, too. Also, quite often, allergic responses diminish when people stop consuming dairy products. For example, a person who is allergic to cats or has asthma symptoms in response to pollen will find that these symptoms diminish when they leave dairy products aside. These are some of the things you can test while you're on the cleanse. If you're ordinarily allergic to cats, for example, you might try being around one while you're off dairy products and see how it goes. I would not, however, advise going off asthma medication without consulting your doctor.

5. Is it safe to do the cleanse when pregnant?

If you are pregnant, dietary advice should come from your physician or obstetrician, with an eye toward any issues that may require special attention. For example, sometimes women run low on iron later in pregnancy, and supplementation would best be customized.

As a general rule during pregnancy, a healthy diet would consist of vegetables, fruits, legumes, and whole grains, and would be certain to include prenatal vitamins, such as B_{12}.

Alcohol is to be entirely avoided during pregnancy, as it is during the cleanse.

I would suggest not going off gluten during pregnancy (unless you have celiac disease, of course), because eating a gluten-free diet can take some getting used to in terms of making sure you are eating a varied diet. [There is an excellent book that addresses this life stage, called *Healthy Eating for Life, for Women.*—KF]

6. I usually eat bran fiber for regularity. Can you suggest a gluten-free substitute that I can use during the cleanse?

If you are eating lots of vegetables and whole grains, you will be getting plenty of naturally occurring fiber. That said, I would add into your daily routine two tablespoons of freshly ground flaxseed. You can sprinkle it over oatmeal or into a salad, or mix it into a smoothie. Flaxseed is not only a great source of fiber but is also quite high in omega-3 fatty acids, which have been shown to lower cholesterol, blood triglycerides, and blood pressure. Regular consumption of flaxseed might also help to prevent a heart attack by keeping the blood platelets from becoming sticky. Flaxseeds also contain something called lignin, which has shown promise in preventing cancer and other diseases.

7. I seem to be a little more bloated than usual on this cleanse. Do you have suggestions on how to reduce bloating?

If the problem is gassiness, beans are a common culprit. They should not be excluded from the diet, however, because they are great sources of protein, calcium, and iron, among other nutrients. But if you are new to beans, it is good to have them in small portions and always very well cooked. A well-cooked bean is soft, with no hint of crunchiness. As time goes on, your digestive tract adjusts, so a bean that may cause a problem today may be better tolerated later on.

Also, cruciferous vegetables can cause indigestion for some people. The answer is simply to cook them well. This group includes broccoli, cauliflower, brussels sprouts, kale, and cabbage, among others. It is common for people to eat them raw or only slightly cooked, but that way can easily cause gassiness or bloating. Cook them well, and the problem usually disappears. Later on, you can experiment again with less-cooked vegetables.

On the good side, rice is easily digested, and a great food to emphasize. Brown rice is best. Also, cooked green, yellow, and orange vegetables are easily digested.

Fruits vary. Some people do well with raw fruit; others have more difficulty at first. If you are new to any particular fruit (and remember to choose ones that are not too sweet), you might have smaller servings at first, then gradually increase.

Sometimes overuse of oils or oily foods can cause bloating, as well. As oils touch the intestinal tract wall, they can disrupt the normally smooth peristaltic movements. So, while the intestinal tract moves its contents along the way a tube of toothpaste is squeezed from one end to the other, oily foods can make it feel like you are squeezing both ends at the same time. So go light on the oil, and stick to the healthier ones, like olive oil and flaxseed oil.

Digestive enzymes can be used, but are usually unnecessary.

8. I notice that rice cakes are included on the shopping list, but I thought they were to be avoided because they are high on the glycemic index. Please explain.

Rice cakes are fine; just keep in mind that they are mostly composed of air. A typical rice cake has only 35 calories, with 7 grams of carbohydrate. While it's true that their GI is moderate to high, depending on the brand, you'll want to remember what the GI represents. When a food's GI is calculated, volunteers consume 50 grams of carbohydrate, and their blood sugar is then tracked over time. It's easy to get 50 grams of carbohydrate from a soda or a piece of cake, but to consume 50 grams of carbohydrate from rice cakes, you would have to eat more than seven full-size rice cakes, which is a far bigger serving than you are likely to eat.

Nutrition researchers believe that the GI is not especially important for foods that are this low in carbohydrate and calories. As they would put it, the glycemic index is moderate to high, but the glycemic load is actually quite low, and that's what counts. Also, common rice cakes are composed of brown rice, so you get fiber as part of it. Of course, having a serving of actual brown rice has advantages over the cakes, but having one or two rice cakes as a snack is perfectly fine. [I like them with a nut butter spread!—*KF*]

9. I heard that eating soy is not good for people, hormonally, and we should stay away from it. Is that true?

Actually, the opposite is true, at least for women. Many studies have looked at this issue, and, in January 2008, University of Southern California researchers summarized the results. It turns out that women who have about one serving of soy products (one cup of soymilk or about one-half cup of tofu) each day have about a 30 percent lower risk of developing breast cancer, compared with women who have little or no soy products in their diets.

The usual explanation for this benefit is that natural compounds in soy products block the effects of a woman's natural estrogens. Normally, the estrogens in a woman's bloodstream attach to receptors protruding from the cells of her body, just as planes at an airport pull up to the Jetways to discharge their passengers. Natural soy compounds adhere to these receptors, blocking the estrogens from attaching. That's a good thing. Estrogens can fuel the growth of cancer cells, and reducing estrogen effects cuts cancer risk. Now, soy's actual effects on cells are probably more complicated than this simple explanation, but it serves to illustrate that soy products are beneficial from the standpoint of cancer prevention. There are fewer studies for women who have already had cancer, but evidence to date suggests no risk from soy.

Studies have also looked at soy's effects on men. There are no adverse hormonal effects. If anything, when soy products replace meat or dairy products, a man is more likely to remain slim and healthy. And don't forget that meaty diets contribute to the artery blockages that not only cause heart disease but also contribute to impotence (without adequate blood flow, an erection is impossible). So having tofu or tempeh instead of meat is likely to help a man remain sexually active as the years go by.

10. How much protein do I actually need, and will I get enough on this cleanse?

Protein comes up as a question all the time, although it is, in fact, a nonissue. But to answer your question, let me list the government's recommended protein intakes. I should mention that health-conscious people should try to stay on the low side of these recommendations and get their protein from plant, rather than animal, sources. Animal protein, among other problems it presents, is associated with osteoporosis and gradual loss of kidney function.

How Much Protein?

The government's nutrition authorities handle this in two ways:

The Recommended Dietary Allowance for adults is 0.8 grams per kilogram of body weight, which works out to 0.36 grams per pound. So, for a person who weighs 150 pounds, that would amount to 54 grams of protein daily. This includes a considerable margin of error, and the actual amount needed may be less than this.

The National Academy of Sciences recommends that protein intake be at least 10 percent of one's daily calories (and no more than 35 percent of daily calories). So let's say a woman consumes 1,800 calories per day. Since a gram of protein has 4 calories, she should be getting at least 45 grams of protein per day ($180 \div 4 = 45$).

What does this look like in food portions? Here are a few examples:

Baked beans (vegetarian), 1 cup:	12.2
Black beans, 1 cup:	15.2
Broccoli, 1 cup:	5.8
Brown rice, 1 cup:	5.0
Oatmeal, 1 cup:	6.1
Peas (green), 1 cup:	8.6
Spaghetti (white), 1 cup:	6.7
Spinach (cooked), 1 cup	5.3
Tofu (firm), ½ cup:	10–20 (depending on type)

The American Dietetic Association and Dietitians of Canada issued a joint statement in 2003 on the adequacy of vegetarian and vegan diets. Here are a few excerpts:

> Well-planned vegan and other types of vegetarian diets are appropriate for all stages of the life cycle, including during pregnancy, lactation, infancy, childhood, and adolescence.

> Research indicates that an assortment of plant foods eaten over the course of a day can provide all essential

amino acids and ensure adequate nitrogen retention and use in healthy adults, thus complementary proteins do not need to be consumed at the same meal.

Athletes can also meet their protein needs on plant-based diets.

With regard to nutrient adequacy, a much more important issue is vitamin B_{12}, which comes most conveniently from a daily multiple vitamin (all brands have B_{12}). This is good advice for anyone, vegetarian or not. The government recently began recommending B_{12} supplements (as opposed to food sources) for everyone over the age of fifty, but a B_{12} supplement is essential for vegans at any age.

11. What are the physical changes I can expect to see upon completion of the cleanse?

You will definitely see changes in the twenty-one days. Weight loss will begin, of course, and can range quite widely, from two to three pounds up to about ten pounds over a three-week period, although it is good to start slowly, around one pound per week. But the 21-Day Cleanse also resets your tastes, so that greasy, unhealthy foods won't call out so insistently, and that means that people who need to lose much more weight are now set to accomplish that. Over the long run, weight loss will be much more profound.

Blood pressure, both systolic and diastolic, usually falls a few points in the first few weeks, and the drop continues if weight loss continues. Eventually, many people taking blood pressure medications are able to discontinue them.

Cholesterol and triglycerides (blood fats) typically fall

by as much as 30 percent in about four weeks' time, although it takes up to twelve weeks to see the full effect of a diet adjustment. Again, many people on cholesterol-lowering drugs can stop them if they stick with a vegan diet.

If a person has diabetes, blood glucose will fall, as will hemoglobin A1c (a test for longer-term blood sugar control). Some people have profound drops in blood glucose within a week or two, although most people need longer—perhaps six months—for the full effect of diet changes to become apparent. Eventually, many people can reduce or even discontinue diabetes medications. It is important to do this only when your doctor says the time is right.

Migraines and arthritis usually go away or improve dramatically. Digestive problems, such as chronic constipation or irritable bowel, usually improve or remit entirely. Sleep is often dramatically better, as is energy.

Over the long run, cancer risk is cut to about half what it was before the diet change.

Sometimes, people who are really hooked on caffeine, sugar, chocolate, alcohol, cheese, and other substances, have a bit of a withdrawal during the first several days, often manifesting as lower mood, lack of energy, or irritability, very much like a smoker who quits. As they come out of that phase, they are glad to have broken free.

Day 14:

The Perfection of a Plant-Based Diet

I THOUGHT I'D TAKE TODAY TO CONTINUE THE DISCUSSION ABOUT protein, because really, it's the single most misunderstood topic and most frequently asked question I get: "How in the world do you get enough protein if you aren't even eating fish or eggs?" It's easy to buy into the protein myth, and I think that has happened in part because of the Atkins diet and heavy promotion by the animal agricultural industries. But there's so much more to the protein story, and a steady stream of research is coming out supporting a plant-based diet and noting the perils of a meat-based one. But the main issue here is that you will find *plenty* of protein on the cleanse; it is not hard to do.

To recap what Dr. Barnard said yesterday, humans need only about 10 percent of the calories we consume to be from protein. Athletes and pregnant women need a little more, but if you're eating enough calories from a varied plant-based diet, it's close to impossible not to get enough.

The way Americans obsess about protein, you'd think

protein deficiency was the number-one health problem in America. The fact is, it's not even on the list of ailments doctors are worried about in America or any other countries where basic caloric needs are being met.

What is on the list? Heart disease, cancer, diabetes, obesity—diseases of affluence. Diseases linked to eating animal products.

Dr. Dean Ornish writes of his "Eat More, Weigh Less" vegetarian diet—the one diet that has passed peer review for taking weight off and keeping it off for more than five years—that in addition to being the one scientifically proven weight-loss plan that works long-term, it "may help to prevent a wide variety of other illnesses including breast cancer in women, prostate cancer in men, colon cancer, lung cancer, lymphoma, osteoporosis, diabetes, hypertension, and so on. . . ."

So when people ask me about protein, I explain that not only is protein not a problem on a vegan diet plan, but the real problems that are plaguing us in the West can be addressed in part by eliminating meat. I get my protein the same way everyone else does—I eat!

Beans, nuts, seeds, lentils, and whole grains are packed with protein. Even vegetables have some protein in them. These protein sources have some excellent benefits that animal protein does not—they contain plenty of fiber and complex carbohydrates, where meat has none. That's right: *meat has no complex carbs at all, and no fiber.* And we need complex (not simple and refined, mind you) carbohydrates to thrive and be healthy. By contrast, plant proteins are packed with these essential nutrients.

Plus, since plant-based protein sources don't contain cholesterol or high amounts of saturated fat, they are much better for you than meat, eggs, and dairy products.

Did You Know?

Olympian Carl Lewis has said that his best year of track competition was the first year that he ate a vegan diet. (He is still a strong proponent of vegan diets for athletes.)

Strength trainer Mike Mahler says, "Becoming a vegan had a profound effect on my training. . . . My bench press excelled past 315 pounds, and I noticed that I recovered much faster. My body fat also went down, and I put on 10 pounds of lean muscle in a few months."

Bodybuilder Robert Cheeke advises, "The basics for nutrition are consuming large amounts of fresh green vegetables and a variety of fruits, to load yourself up with vibrant vitamins and minerals."

Other vegans, who sing the praises of the diet for their athletic performance include: ultimate fighter Mac Danzig, ultramarathoner Scott Jurek, Minnesota Twins pitcher Pat Neshek, Atlanta Hawks guard Salim Stoudamire, and Kansas City Chiefs tight end Tony Gonzalez.

And let's not forget about basketball's all-time great John Salley, tennis star Martina Navratilova, six-time Ironman winner Dave Scott, four-time Mr. Universe Bill Pearl, or Stan Price, the world-record holder in bench press. They are just a few of the successful vegetarian athletes.

Vegans and vegetarians needn't fret about protein, but many of us do need to worry about our weight, heart disease, cancer, and other ailments—many of which can be addressed by exactly the kind of eating you are doing on your cleanse. So keep it up and delight in the fact that you are temporarily disengaging from all those foods that have been dragging your body down.

Today's Meditation

I ease into a new way of being. I can relax knowing that my decision to eat a plant-based diet is well researched and sound. I have been moving toward the notion of conscious eating for many reasons, and I find myself at this place with a willing and open mind. It is a relief to know that science backs up what I instinctively felt. The earth, with all its abundant riches, provides for me everything I need. I am becoming more aligned and in sync with the natural and benevolent flow of life. I may not know everything there is to know yet, but my mind is open and I am willing to keep leaning in to this shift that I know is taking me to a higher stage of awareness and living. I ease into it, trusting that this is exactly where I am supposed to be.

Week Three

DAY 15:

The Ripple Effect

TWO OUT OF THE THREE WEEKS ARE BEHIND YOU NOW. I BOW to your strength. You took such a leap by cutting out all that in one big swoop. But please remember: if you slip, it's okay. As you know by now, my whole approach to health and wellness is that it's about leaning toward change and taking small steps to support growth; there is no need to force yourself into something that is terribly uncomfortable. Just lean.

I advocate this gentle approach to just about every kind of change we choose to make in life. We show up, do the best we can, and take baby steps until we feel comfortable taking bigger steps or embracing the change wholeheartedly. Of course, if you're a single parent or are holding down an excessively busy job, you may have to compromise in some ways; that's okay—you're doing the best you can, which is all anyone can ask.

Just staying awake and aware of where your food comes from and how you feel when you eat it is such a big step in the right direction. This awareness alone is enough to kick off a momentum that I promise you *will not stop*. Once you're paying attention, it's hard to go back to sleep.

Among the many quotes that I love from Martin Luther King Jr. is this: "One of the great liabilities of history is that all too many people fail to remain awake through great periods of social change. But today our very survival depends on our ability to stay awake, to adjust to new ideas, to remain vigilant and face the challenge of change." As seductive as it is, then, to drift off to sleep, we simply can't. Now, more than ever, we have to pay attention.

If you look around our world today, there are so many things that seem to have gotten to a critical point. One of them is the environment. Never in human history has the planetary condition been so dire: polar ice caps are melting, bringing ocean levels up to the point where flooding is inevitable. Large chunks of land are disappearing. The water is warming, killing countless species of fish and coral, and allowing suffocating algae to flourish and create "dead zones"—miles and miles of ocean that can no longer sustain life. The warming of the earth's atmosphere is causing increasingly numerous and fierce storms, which pose relentless threats to coastal cities and towns that are situated next to major rivers. Other parts of the world, such as Africa, are suffering severe drought and food shortage; and places like where I live in California are experiencing devastating cycles of wildfires and ensuing mudslides. (With the disappearance of trees and brush due to fire, the earth is far more susceptible to mudslides.)

It's hard to remain asleep when it seems like life itself is shaking us to wake up and do things differently. As Dr.

King sagely cautioned, our survival is at stake. This is no time to kick back and enjoy the "bliss" of ignorance. In fact, this is the time to rise to our full capacity to become the change agents that this world so sorely needs by being mindful about how we consume. In every little choice we make of what to buy, which industry to support or not support, we make a difference.

A Few Facts About Eating an Animal-Free, Plant-Based Diet

Some of the following facts will make you feel even better about your choice to try an animal-free, plant-based diet.

According to United Nations scientists in a recent 408-page scientific analysis of raising animals in order to eat them, eating meat, dairy, and eggs is "one of the . . . most significant contributors to the most serious environmental problems at every scale from local to global" and "should be a major policy focus when dealing with problems of land degradation, climate change and air pollution, water shortage and water pollution, and loss of biodiversity." Please read that again, it's pretty stunning! Here's why:

> **Land degradation:** More than 90 percent of the Amazon rain forest cleared since 1970, or about 45,000 square miles, is now being used by the meat industry, either for grazing or to grow crops to feed farmed animals. That forest is like a giant sink that holds in carbon dioxide. When it is cut down or burned, the carbon dioxide is released in massive

amounts, thus contributing to global warming. And here in our country, 260 million acres of our forests have been cleared to grow crops to feed farmed animals as well.

Climate change: Animal agriculture causes almost 40 percent more greenhouse gas emissions than all the cars, trucks, and planes in the world combined. (That figure just shocked me.) The digestive processes of farmed animals (including their excrement, which is 130 times that produced by the U.S. human population), combine to release staggering amounts of carbon dioxide, methane, and nitrous oxide into the atmosphere. The carbon footprint of processing animal foods is far higher than that of plant foods because of the additional energy-intensive steps: processing and shipping feed crops, slaughtering animals, dismembering and processing their bodies, freezing their bodies for shipment, etc. All this requires an awful lot of oil and electricity. The Environmental Defense Fund explains, "If every American skipped one meal of chicken per week and substituted vegetables and grains, for example, the carbon dioxide savings would be the same as taking more than half a million cars off U.S. roads." So celebrate the good you're doing by eating chicken-free for three entire weeks!

Air pollution: In Texas alone, feedlots produce more than 14 million pounds of particulate dust, which "contains biologically active organisms such as bacteria, mold, and fungi from the feces and the feed." The California State Senate reports: "studies have also shown that [animal waste] lagoons emit toxic airborne chemicals that can cause inflammatory, immune, irritation, and neurochemical problems in humans." On top of that, the EPA has found that 80 percent of the toxic ammonia gas in the United States comes from farmed animal excrement. It is said that if you walk into one of these huge factory farms, the ammonia nearly knocks you off your feet and it's nearly impossible to breathe without your lungs burning. *New Yorker* reporter Michael Specter visited a chicken shed in Maryland and described the experience this way: "I was almost knocked to the ground by the overpowering smell of feces and ammonia. My eyes burned and so did my lungs, and I could neither see nor breathe."

Water shortage and pollution: Animal agriculture is one of the main causes of water shortage in the western United States, in that it requires between three and eleven times the water required to grow an equal amount of soy. Copious amounts are needed to raise feed crops, provide animals drinking water, and wash away feces and urine. The runoff from factory farms is laced with feces, bacteria, hormones, and antibiotics, which can dangerously affect our arable soil and potable drinking water. The high levels of nitrogen from the animal feces along with the crop fertilizers (most crops are fed to farmed animals) devastates life in local waterways by promoting algae blooms, thus creating the aforementioned "dead zones."

Loss of biodiversity: As more land is used for grazing and to grow feed crops, native birds and mammals are pushed to the brink. In addition, the oceans are being devastated by commercial fishing. A recent alarming study found that 90 percent of large fish populations have been exterminated in the past fifty years because of large-scale fishing. In many areas, it's like clear-cutting the ocean floor. Fish farming just exacerbates the problem, as ocean fish are caught and fed to fish in fish farms. It takes several pounds of ocean-caught fish to produce a pound of farmed fish flesh.

There's more . . .

There is an ever-increasing and persistent problem of hunger in some developing nations, so that currently, more than 850 million people are starving, and tens of millions die annually from starvation-related causes. An enormous amount of corn, soy, and grain—crops that could feed humans and keep them from starving—is being diverted to feed farm animals. Here's the problem: eating meat requires that we feed animals first, and most of what we feed to them they don't turn into meat—they burn it up just existing. So it turns out that 760 million tons of grain are fed to chickens, pigs, and cattle every year. You might well imagine how many hungry people all that grain could satisfy were it not going to the more high-paying wealthy industries of factory farming. Poor people are now in competition with factory farms for food!

Look at it this way: the amount of feed that it takes to funnel through an animal to create one 8-ounce steak could fill forty to fifty bowls with cooked grain. The *Independent* (a UK paper), recently cited that "while 100 million tons of grain are being diverted to make fuel this year, over seven times as much (760 million tons) will be used to feed animals. The world's passion for meat is a much bigger cause of global hunger than its passion for the car." Let that one sink in for a minute: "the world's passion for meat is . . . a cause of global hunger."

Clearly, eating animal protein has gotten out of hand. Formerly a garnish, or a once-in-a-while special meal, meat, eggs, and dairy have become the mainstay of Western diets (and sadly, now our diet has spread to nearly every corner of the world). We eat over 50 percent more meat today than we did in 1950, and four times as much poultry. It's this voracious appetite for meat—driven by clever marketing and animal agriculture's insatiable grab for profit—that has given rise to enormous factory farms. Small family-owned farms are nearly extinct, and although there is a rising interest in locally grown food, it's the factory farms that process the vast majority of animals. So every time we say "no thank you" to a turkey sandwich or steak dinner, we are withholding our money and support from an industry that has the single most deleterious effect on the environment of all industries. And as our families and friends begin to see the wisdom of our choices, they, too, might explore the possibility of eating more responsibly.

Amazing, isn't it, that a food choice can carry so much weight? Truly, everything is connected. What's good for one aspect of our well-being—our physical health—is also good for others, as in planetary well-being. By choosing to eat healthfully, we are not only doing a good thing for ourselves, but we are also benefiting the natural world with all its interconnecting ecosystems.

Helpful Tip

If people roll their eyes or give you a hard time about not eating meat, tell them you are doing the most powerful thing you can do for the environment by abstaining from meat, fish, dairy, and eggs. Let them know that "Vegetarian is the new Prius!" Buying a hybrid car is a great thing to do, but not everyone can afford one, and it's a one-time deal. By eating a plant-based diet, even for just these twenty-one days, you are making a positive choice not just for yourself but also for the repair of the world.

Today's Meditation

I make a difference. With every choice we make, we are shepherding our energy—our values and beliefs—out into the world. We are exerting our power by saying no to industries that cause so much harm. By educating (with kindness) our families, friends, and coworkers, our choices ripple out and have an ever-widening and far-reaching effect. We are creating the future as we go, and that is serious, and empowering, business. *I make a difference*, and today, I take pride in that.

Day 16:

Coming out of the Sugar Slump

Back to the Big Five. The last of the Big Five, I might add.

Of the many things we can do to improve our health, regulating and/or cutting down on our daily sugar intake is certainly one of the most important. Our bodies are not genetically set up to handle high amounts of sugars and refined carbohydrates; many different kinds of diseases can develop from the imbalance "oversugaring" brings about. That's why it's one of the Big Five foods you are staying away from for the duration of the cleanse.

Sugar is not in and of itself a bad thing. Basically, sugar is the body's primary source of fuel. In the proper amounts and from a natural, unrefined source, glucose is beneficial and necessary for health, and even life. But in our modern diet we go far beyond what is required and give the body too much of a necessary thing and also a lot of what's not necessary at all.

Keep in mind that we get all the sugar we need from a

natural diet. Plant foods—including grains—have a certain amount of sugar in them. When we eat them, our digestive process breaks down the food and makes the glucose available to our cells. So sugar is not something that must be added to an already healthy diet. It need not be a supplement.

The World Health Organization released dietary guidelines in 2003 that stated that not more than 10 percent of your total overall diet should come from sugar. The average energy requirement is two thousand calories per day, so that means that no more than two hundred calories, or about 50 grams, should be from simple sugars. Bear in mind that 10 percent is the upper limit, sort of like a speed limit. It's not a place to begin but a boundary beyond which you can do yourself harm.

The sugar industry lobby, of course, refutes that and says up to 25 percent is okay. To me, that's like the oil industry claiming that it's better for traffic if people drive more.

As an example of how much sugar is in an ordinary food, take a look at yogurt. The average serving of low-fat yogurt contains about 32 grams of sugar, which is the equivalent of eight teaspoons. That means that in one fairly small portion of a "healthy" food you've consumed about 64 percent of the total daily recommended sugar intake. You can see how easy it is to go beyond that, especially with fruit or soda drinks, anything with corn syrup (which is added to countless processed foods and even to a lot of deli items you'd never suspect), and refined carbs like white bread or conventional cereal.

Consider This:

By now you might have noticed that your stomach is slightly flatter. That's what not having any sugar or gluten can do. Eating sugar contributes to an overgrowth of a fungus in the body. This fungus is called *Candida albicans*, and along with being a factor in causing excess infections (bladder, yeast, etc.), it can cause gas, irritable bowel, and fluid retention. On the mental plane, it also brings about fatigue and anxiety. And this yeast craves things that will make it thrive, so the more yeast you have in your body, the more you will crave alcohol, sweets, and processed, bready foods. It's sort of like a creature that lives inside of you, forcing you to eat more of the stuff that will "feed the beast." This is why it's so important not to give in to the impulse to binge on conventional desserts and sugary snacks; if you give in, you feed the yeasty beast and make it all the harder to move away from old habits.

Sugar-Based Health Conditions

There are a number of terms that refer to health problems that are sugar-based. Insulin resistance, glucose intolerance, type 2 diabetes, metabolic syndrome: all are conditions that are telling us that the body's basic energy processing is dangerously out of balance. To oversimplify it just a bit, when we eat, a certain amount of insulin corresponding with the sugar level in the food is released by the body so that the glucose can be metabolized and used as energy. But if we eat overly sweet foods as a habit, over time the insulin becomes less effective and glucose is either stored as fat or stays in the system: the body's blood sugar levels rise and stay high, leading to all kinds of health problems associated with type 2 diabetes, or sustained high blood sugar.

Adult-onset diabetes, or type 2, is the most common form of diabetes. With type 2, your body has either stopped producing enough insulin or your cells are desensitized to it (that's what is known as insulin resistance).

Insulin resistance and type 2 diabetes are problems that creep up on many people; they don't realize how sick they are until it's too late and their health is in a dangerous state. But there are warning signs to look for along the way. The most basic one is general fatigue. Being tired all the time can have many causes, of course, but if you're getting at least seven hours of sleep per night, you should look at your blood sugar levels. Another warning sign is mental confusion and the inability to concentrate. Still others are weight gain (especially around your middle), sleeplessness, loss of circulation (a cold feeling) in your outer limbs. These all can be signs of being on the road to type 2 diabetes. You'll need a doctor's blood sugar test to confirm this, though.

It is said that sugar "feeds" cancer. This is because one of the things that insulin does is promote cell growth, and if you have cancer cells in your body, sugar can act like fertilizer on them. The more insulin you have in your body (remember, it is released in response to ingesting sugar or the like), the more cancer cells can proliferate. The good news is that simple changes, like switching from regular sodas to sparkling water with lime, or stevia-sweetened treats instead of sugary ones, will often lead you back to health. Try them and see how you feel, at least for these twenty-one days. If you don't feel a whole lot better by removing sugar from your diet, then most definitely see a doctor. Even if you are not insulin resistant, it's a good idea to stick to healthier sweeteners if you want to be slim, healthy, and even-keeled with your energy.

Aside from eating less sugar, exercise is crucial for people who are prediabetic (those on the road to type 2 diabetes). This is because physical activity forces the body to use its stored-up glucose as energy, rather than allowing it to build up in the body and cause damage throughout.

Though it hasn't been conclusively proven, sugar is clearly addictive for many people, or has addictive properties. How many of us get intense cravings for sweet foods and refined carbs like pasta? In fact, sugar often increases the appetite. This function of sweet foods was a healthy response when calories were scarce and it was necessary to eat as much as possible while food was available. But our modern lives do not need this extra urging; we have as much food as we need at all times. So we are stuck with this response from sweet foods: eat more of them whether or not we need the calories (and we don't).

Some people who are addicted to sugar feel physically unwell most of the time. They may not even realize that they feel bad until they kick sugar and suddenly feel well; they had become habituated to feeling lethargic because they have nothing much to compare it to, other than that very temporary "high" they feel for a few minutes at a time after ingesting something sugary. That's an example of how the insulin spike works: you eat something sweet and have some immediate energy, but soon that wears off and you are left feeling wasted, often far worse than before you ate the thing with a high sugar content. If that's your entire life, as it is for far too many of us, this cleanse will be like an awakening for you.

What to Expect as You Kick Your Sugar Habit

I will admit, it's not easy to quit sugar. Though it's not considered a drug like nicotine or opium, I sometimes think it should be, since some people do experience withdrawal symptoms when they stop ingesting it. For those who are affected, sugar withdrawal can include headaches, dizziness, irritability, and fatigue. Along with that, sugar addicts will crave it even more than before. This is because their bodies are out of balance and they have taken away the fuel for the imbalance. It can take a few days or even a week to regain metabolic harmony.

People get sugar cravings for a number of reasons. First off, ingesting sugar can temporarily increase levels of serotonin, which can make you feel good, but only for a short time. Second, sweet foods are often used as a reward or in times of stress, a soother to make you feel better, so there is a psychological component to the cycle.

Another reason you might crave sweets is because of insulin resistance. As your body stops being able to use insulin effectively, glucose is turned into fat instead of used as fuel. Your cells, deprived of fuel, signal to your body that they need more, and you get cravings for more foods rich in glucose, which still can't be utilized and is stored as fat, thus depriving your cells, which send out more cravings . . . and the cycle continues.

As noted, most people won't have physical withdrawal problems from stopping sugar consumption, but if you do, within a few days of starting the cleanse, your metabolism will begin to rebalance and you will cease experiencing that insatiable longing for sugar. In fact, as you decrease and finally cut out sugars altogether, your body's energy will slowly come back into harmony because you are no longer feeding the two main culprits of sugar-caused imbalance, type 2 diabetes (continual high blood sugar) and hypo-glycemia (low blood sugar brought on by a spike in insulin in reaction to a high sugar intake). And in the case of hypoglycemia, your adrenal glands will get some relief, because they no longer have to compensate for low blood sugar levels. In the case of type 2 diabetes, even in its pre-diabetic stage, your body will be able to begin using the glucose in the blood for energy instead of storing it as fat. Either way, your energy levels will pick up and maintain in a steady way.

Your job over these twenty-one days is to become aware of sugar levels in foods, even foods you wouldn't suspect, and to understand that you really don't need any added sugar whatsoever to get enough for your body's natural needs. If you do find yourself wanting sugar, try eating a piece of fruit or drink a glass of water with a dash of lemon. But the most important thing to realize is that no matter how out of balance your system is, even if you have type 2 diabetes, you can do a great deal to get healthy again by cutting out sugars, refined carbs, and high-fructose corn syrup, and by exercising regularly.

In short, continue to avoid:

- Soda
- **Store-bought cookies, cakes, or pastries**
- **Fruit juice (even though juice sounds natural, it contains high concentrations of naturally occurring sugar, and should be generally avoided)**
- **Candy**
- **Condiments that contain sugar or high fructose corn syrup (HFCS)**
- **High-glycemic fruits, such as watermelon, mango, or pineapple (a simple Internet search will yield lists of high-glycemic and low-glycemic foods)**
- **Maple syrup, honey, sugar, chemical sugar substitutes (such as Splenda, Equal, Sweet'n Low)**
- **Ice cream or frozen yogurt**

Here is just a partial list of all the sweet foods you can enjoy:

- **Fruits such as Granny Smith apples, blueberries, or cherries**
- **Water or sparkling water with a squeeze of lemon or lime**
- **Homemade or health-food store goodies that are sweetened only with stevia, xylitol, or**

agave (some people don't do well with agave, so proceed with caution).

The Lean

Although this is a cleanse and it's fairly important to keep the Big Five out of your diet in as pure a way as possible, I also realize that we are human and therefore will not be perfect all the time. That's okay. If, for instance, there is a smidge of sweetener that you had not at first noticed in a loaf of bread you found in the health food store, go ahead and enjoy it. The cleanse is not about deprivation, but rather about creating an awareness around food and how it affects your body. Do the best you can and keep moving forward.

DAY 17:

Choose Wisely

BY NOW THE CLEANSE HAS PROBABLY TAKEN ON A MOMENTUM all its own. You may have noticed that your taste buds have already changed. You no longer crave the Big Five—at least not in the same intense way. In fact, you may already be at the point where you find it hard to believe you were so attached to any of them at all! Your energy has already picked up, and you've lost some weight and gained some muscle. But most of all, you are probably feeling a great sense of personal power and inner alignment in knowing that you have successfully challenged yourself to leave old patterns behind.

Consider This:

People tend to make choices on the basis of two fundamental survival instincts: the desire for pleasure and the avoidance of pain. As we navigate our lives, we are constantly weighing consequences, deciding what's more important to us, and then pushing ourselves to do the thing that will most benefit us. And as far as survival instincts go, the strongest of the two is the avoidance of pain. If, for instance, we don't want to be hit by an oncoming car or get an expensive ticket, we will pay heed to traffic lights and stop signs. By the same token, we choose not to steal because we don't want to get caught and then be punished or humiliated. We make these choices to avoid pain. Morals and ethics, of course, play a part as well. ("I want to be a good, law-abiding citizen, and it is not right to steal or run lights.") In that same vein, we keep up personal hygiene—brushing our teeth, taking showers, using deodorant—not only to stay healthy and smell good but also because we don't want to be thought of as unkempt or unattractive. It's sometimes a chore to "do the right thing," but we do it because it pays off.

Eating well and taking care of our health are sort of the same thing, but we've somehow lost sight of the consequences—the pain—of not making good choices. Probably because many of the consequences are long-term, we often don't feel them immediately (or don't connect the dots if we do). It's instantly gratifying, for instance, to eat some cookies or ice cream because, well, we've had a hard day and they taste good, and it's fun to indulge. We reason to ourselves (in a split-second, unconscious thought process) that everyone else is downing a few beers and shoveling in the chicken wings, so why not just let go and enjoy. Life is for living, right?

The problem here is that while we're right—cookies and the like do taste good—we aren't fully focusing on the future consequences (weight gain, digestive problems, diabetes, heart troubles, etc.), and therefore we aren't calibrating our motivations and actions *today* so that we actually do have the best shot at health and happiness in the long term. Here's an exercise that will help you do just that.

Think About This

Take a look at the joys and consequences of doing things the way you always have, and see if it's worth it to continue.

The pros of eating my favorite foods, like burgers or cookies or fast food, or drinking whatever I feel like are:

- It's fun.
- It takes my mind off the conflict (or monotony) of the moment.
- It tastes good.
- I feel a sense of camaraderie with my friends; I enjoy the social rituals.
- It's easy and convenient.

The cons of eating unhealthily are:

- I only have a quick blast of energy, then I get sluggish and feel tired.
- Over time, I gain weight and have a dull pallor to my skin.
- I always feel slightly guilty and mad at myself for not being healthier.
- My chances of getting cancer, heart disease, and diabetes are greatly increased (by up to 80 percent) by ingesting all that sugar,

alcohol, refined carbohydrates, and animal protein.

- Being ill is terrifying and painful, and once disease is set in motion it takes an enormous amount of effort to turn it around.
- Getting sick is expensive, and my insurance doesn't cover much of it. I can lose much of the wealth that I have worked hard for just in paying health-care bills.
- I feel bloated and uncomfortable.
- I'm not being exemplary to my kids or peers. Rather than breaking away from the pack and being a leader, I am just meandering along with the masses.
- Because so much of what I eat gets me into a cycle of craving and addiction, much of my mental focus goes toward fighting the urge, then succumbing, and then beating myself up. I hardly have anything left over for creativity, inspiration, or being present for all the little wonders of life.
- Since my hormonal chemistry is thrown out of balance by much of the Big Five, I'm moody and don't feel as vibrant as I'd like. I don't feel good about myself or my life.
- I don't feel sexy or attractive, so I shut down to my relationship potential.

Was that cake after dinner worth the consequences? Really, was it?

I bet not.

We pay a big price for momentary gustatory pleasure. If we get into the habit of thinking three steps ahead, we can avoid a lot of pain (both emotional and physical), such as low self-esteem, compromised energy, and endless annoyances and trials with our health. And if we can just get through the temporary discomfort of not having what we want when we want it, there is a big payoff: we are freed from the addictive cycle of craving and guilt, we look and feel both physically and emotionally great, and we save a lot of time, money, and anguish not being sick.

Yes, there is that initial sacrifice of the good and familiar taste; you won't be able to turn to the exact comforts and pleasures you once enjoyed. But you will replace those joys with healthier ones. They may not be quite as delicious or satisfying at first, but with a bit of acclimation, they will become so. Have you ever gone from whole milk to skim milk? For a while, skim seems watery and unsubstantial, but very soon you prefer it, finding whole milk to be way too thick and weighty; this is, as far as I can tell, a universal experience with milk, and it applies every bit as much to the shifts you can make during (and after, if you wish) the cleanse. (This is not to recommend skim milk, by the way; it's only to remind you that new tastes take some time to get used to.)

Although changing our diet is not a breeze, it certainly is worth it—in just about every respect of body, mind, and spirit. It does require that we look at our choices and weigh out the benefits versus what we have to forgo. For me, paying attention to some basic rationale put me over the edge.

Eating a cleaner, more plant-based diet, I realized, was not only good for me on a purely healthy level, it also had important ripple effects and kept me in alignment with my higher values (more on this soon).

While you're on the cleanse, this kind of deep consideration can be very useful in motivating you to stay on course. When you look at how good you can feel by choosing—even if only for three weeks—to opt out of a system where you're a slave to your food, rather than the master of it, coupled with the promise of better health, it's easier to say, "Just for today, I will not bow to my cravings. I can choose something healthier that I will grow to love. I'm leaning in to new ways."

Helpful Tip

At the moment you feel you might cave and scrap the cleanse, remind yourself that you have free will and it is your choice to have or do whatever you want. And then say to yourself, "Okay, I can have this piece of cake [or jigger of Scotch or chunk of cheese, or what have you], but if I do, these are the consequences." And then list them.

Use your rational mind and make smart decisions. Then go and find a delicious substitute!

Today's Meditation

I choose wisely. I am more than just a body on autopilot. I am a thinking, rational, strong person who has pointed myself in the direction of ever-evolving wellness. I am no longer willing to do things just because they feel superficially or temporarily good. I want to experience a deeper sense of satisfaction now, which includes being responsible to myself and to the world around me. I know that sweating it through this period of discomfort will pay off. I know what's right—spiritually and materially—and I'm willing to sacrifice a bit to do it. *I choose wisely*, and with each day, that wisdom lifts me to a higher level.

Day 18:

Addressing the Real Hunger

WITH ANY MOVE TOWARD HEALING, A KEY COMPONENT OF THE process is to engage ourselves at the deepest levels of our being. We are aiming not only to purify the body but also to undertake an inner purification, to move away from our baser instincts so that we may embody our more divine nature.

To forgo immediate gratification (indulging in favorite foods or drinks) in the spirit of experiencing a deeper sort of nourishment is to overcome the self that acted on rote in favor of the Self that thrives on being good, true, and beautiful. Right living requires that we strive to refrain from negative impulses that are self-harming or that harm others, while simultaneously realizing that we can't be perfect and that we should not hide behind that fact; we should do the best we can. On the outside, it may look as if we are sacrificing our tastes and cravings and favorite foods—and in a way, we sometimes are—but the payoff is that we are ratcheting ourselves up the next step of the evolutionary ladder.

If you look at the wise sages throughout history, they

were not bound by a greediness for food, or an insatiable taste for alcohol or coffee. They were not gluttonous. They abstained from certain foods (e.g., alcohol, animal foods) so they could fulfill their aim of becoming enlightened, liberated from violent or self-centered superficial needs. And in a small way, this is what we are learning to do with this 21-Day Cleanse.

We are essentially dropping old preoccupations that would reinforce a stagnant lifestyle in favor of an expanded evolutionary path. But to do this, we have to find new ways to get our needs met. Of course the obvious thing to do is to put only healthy things into our bodies—foods that taste good but that do no harm to ourselves or anyone else. But above and beyond that, we have to find ways to restore ourselves in deeper, more thoughtful ways. We have to begin to realize that our deepest well-being emerges from being less concerned with just ourselves and more concerned with the well-being of others, and the whole. We are shifting our attention away from addictive eating and drinking and learning how to feel filled up by an interconnectedness with all life. The way you get there is to do things that connect you to Spirit.

No matter what your religious affiliation might be, or whether or not you formally embrace a set of rituals or form of worship, I think we can all agree that while we are powerful, we are not all-powerful. Whatever force it is that propels the universe forward, it is the same force that moves through our lives and urges us to grow and expand. And that's what spirituality is all about—connecting with that force that propels the universe forward and deeper—and it is a vital part of living a full life.

Even those of us who would say we are not religious, per se, can recognize that we are connected to some sort of deep and unified source, which I call Spirit. Throughout my life, I have learned and relearned that if I don't maintain a spiritual practice, my ego tends to take over and I begin to feel separate and disconnected from people and the world. I begin to get lost in fears and anxieties because I think everything is up to me to figure out. When I remember that there is something bigger in play than just my little dramas, it's as if air and light are breathed into my tight thinking. I expand rather than contract. Let's consider what it means to *you* to connect to and nurture that something bigger. How do we transcend the narrow focus of "me and mine" and widen the circle of our consideration and understanding?

For many of us, it's through spiritual practice—from conventional church or temple, to yoga, to mindful contemplation—that we continually refocus ourselves on our better nature.

Whether we choose to attend services at a formal house of worship, study with a teacher, join a meditation group, or read intently to learn more of a particular tradition or philosophy, through spiritual practice we increase our capacity to love and be kind, both to ourselves and to others. We learn to think and act out of love, rather than fear. We move from indifference to compassion. And as we lend ourselves to the shift that comes with spiritual practice, we nurture the light inherent within us so that we can then shine that light out into the world. We are aided immeasurably by putting ourselves in the atmosphere of constant coaching.

A Few Questions to Consider

Asking yourself the following questions can help you gain the most from whatever path you choose:

- What are my guiding principles, or spiritual values?
- How could I best put them into practice?
- What in my life isn't in alignment with my values?
- Where can I go or what can I do to feel in touch with Spirit?
- What might be a good way for me to infuse my life with some spirituality?

As you ponder these questions, know that the purpose of our lives is to grow and expand, and to feel ever more connected and at one with the wholeness of which we are all part. Our careers, health challenges, relationships, and everyday happenings are simply the frictions that spur us to become more in touch with our inner selves, the part of us that is pure and raw. And as we do that, we evolve. We lean in to our better selves, until we are ready for the next push.

Exercise

Decide now what you will do to instill or develop a sense of spirituality in your life. If you are too vague in your plan, nothing will change. You might decide to join a regular meditation group or attend a weekly inspirational lecture. You might take daily walks among the trees and think about your place in the universe. Just consider the following when choosing where to go, from *A Course in Miracles*: "A church that does not inspire love has a hidden altar that is not serving the purpose for which Spirit intended it." And then just listen to your inner voice, which will always tell you if a particular teaching is right or not.

Helpful Tip

Remember the importance of little things—remember how you feel when someone cuts you off in line, or drives aggressively, or behaves rudely to you. And remember how you feel when you encounter someone who is light and caring, who does you a small favor. Remember the ripple effects of your behavior, both positive and negative. We can be lights to others, with very little effort, and the practical positive effects can be far beyond anything that is obvious to us.

Remember also that if something is not going to matter to you in thirty minutes, it shouldn't matter to you now. Will you even recall the person who didn't say please or thank you an hour from now? Don't allow small things to bring out any unkindness in you.

Throughout the day, in every decision you make, ask yourself what your highest Self would do. If you were already completely enlightened, how would you handle things? How would you respond? What energy would you extend? And then act as if you were that person.

Today's Meditation

I am aligned with Spirit. I see that life is about more than just what meets the eye. I am supposed to lift myself, every day, in small ways and significant ones. When I don't quite know what or how to be, I simply imagine myself filled with light and then act in the way that best translates that light. If I am troubled, I step out of my ego—my controlling nature—and surrender the details to Spirit. I know that grace is all around me, assisting me in finding my higher nature.

Day 19:

Divinization

Today, there are no exercises or tips, just one important question to contemplate: How are we to heal, to progress?

A question I am often asked is, What exactly do you mean by "quantum wellness" and what are the most important messages of the book? To me, quantum wellness means that health and happiness can be achieved on an enormous scale by doing small and almost imperceptible things. That a leap from *A* all the way to *Z* can happen if we simply agitate the status quo, and keep agitating. That even one tiny shift in the way we live can ripple out to create far-reaching cultural change in a manner we might never imagine.

Just as the great scientists note in their experiments in quantum physics, we don't know exactly *how* the leap occurs, but we do know it has a lot to do with where the observer puts her attention. So, quantum wellness is largely about *attention*, or awareness.

Rather than insisting on a strict and particular discipline for living, I find great inspiration in Gandhi's thinking on the question of how we should lead our lives. Gandhi called his autobiography his "experiment in truth." He told his followers that he was simply doing the best he could, and that people should take or leave the things he wrote or said on the basis of their own experiences. He challenges all of us to do the best we can in our lives, leading lives of thoughtfulness and striving to do better tomorrow than we did today. In my mind, that means "progress, not perfection."

Going much farther back, more than two millennia earlier, Socrates argued that "the unexamined life is not worth living." It makes sense to me that we are called to examine our lives, to consider who we are, and why we are, and what we're doing.

Sadly, that's not what our culture usually wants of us— our culture wants us to listen to Madison Avenue, not to our hearts and minds, and certainly not to our inner voice of compassion and unity. And sadly, Madison Avenue has ulterior motives—they want to sell us things, generally things we don't need. The job of Madison Avenue is to persuade us into believing that we're not good enough without the latest beauty product, clothing, or gadget—something we've never heard of suddenly becomes something we can't live without, courtesy of the great power of advertising.

But the promise of quantum wellness challenges us to consider health and happiness not as something that is finite or that can be compartmentalized, not as something that just involves our physical health, or just involves our emotional health, or just involves our spiritual health. Quantum wellness encompasses our whole being. We are called to be integrally healthful, and it appears to be a rule of the universe that if something is good for us in one area (i.e., if it's good for our spirit . . .), it is good for us in all areas (. . . it will also be good for our body). And of course the reverse is also true.

The iconoclastic French Jesuit Pierre Teilhard de Chardin brought a twentieth-century outlook to the question of examined lives, challenging us not just to examine our lives but also to focus them on creating a greater world. I agree with his principal point that the goal of humanity and all human beings is to ask ourselves this: "Gloriously situated by life at this critical point in the evolution of humankind, what ought we to do? We hold Earth's future in our hands. What shall we decide?"

Great question. This moment in our lives, and every moment, is potentially transformative. What shall we decide?

The mathematical cosmologist Brian Swimme puts the pieces together for us, explaining that for Teilhard, "by learning to see, by becoming alert and awake in this universe, you feel the call and the presence of the unborn God asking for, or guiding us into, the type of creative action that gives birth to the next moment in a process that [Teilhard] called *'divinization'*" or human participation in creating the better world that is inevitably coming.

Gandhi, Socrates, Teilhard, and other great thinkers challenge us to live examined lives, to make our decisions— from the smallest and most mundane to, of course, the largest and most life-changing—with our eyes wide open, *consciously* focusing on what we're doing and not doing, and why, rather than simply doing what comes next. These great thinkers challenge us to lead our lives as our own "experiments in truth," focused both on awareness and on creating a better world.

The best part is that if we lead "examined lives," if our "experiment in truth" is focused on making the world kinder, if we participate in Teilhard's "divinization" of the world around us, that will also be the best thing for us—spiritually, emotionally, and physically. In leading lives for the greater good, we find our true selves and we find inspiration and empowerment—the self-actualization discussed by psychologist Abraham Maslow as the pinnacle on our hierarchy of needs.

What to figure out for ourselves, then, is this: how can we lead lives that feel fulfilling, healthy, and abundant, with the overarching aim of participating in the divinization Teilhard discussed? Here is the secret: divinization, or the process of bringing light into the world, is both the means and the end. It is a high and noble goal, of course, but it is the pursuit of it that brings us the deepest and most fulfilling joy. By lending ourselves to this great task of enlightenment (for ourselves and the world we live in), we position ourselves right in the vortex of creation itself.

This personal and then global transformation is what will make us feel more whole, more plugged in, and immensely powerful.

So how do we set this process in motion? First off, we address the things that keep us from living fully conscious lives. By looking at where we may be asleep (eating without thinking of where our food comes from, for example, or blindly reenacting old patterns of relating learned from childhood), we open up to greater awareness which allows us to know ourselves—and in turn, to know others—more fully. This kind of deep understanding creates empathy and has us feeling more connected and insightful, more willing and able to be the connective fiber that draws together all the broken and wounded bits in ourselves and in those we come in contact with. As we extend this sort of reparative energy past ourselves and into the world, we fulfill our ultimate purpose and potential of Teilhard's divinization. We become healers, bringers of light.

Let's break it down. Within our relationships—spouses, friends, and work associates—we can push ourselves to realize that we are not so unlike each other. We can remind ourselves that everyone has desires for their lives and the world that are remarkably similar to those we have, even when it's not immediately apparent in an unpleasant interaction. We can forgive ourselves by making amends when they are necessary, taking responsibility for causing pain and then making adjustments so that we don't do it again. We can systematically question what drives us, and then pause before acting without kindness. And we can forgive others by letting them know, when appropriate, how and why they hurt us, requesting that they please refrain from doing it again.

The task in this work of amends and forgiveness, of letting go of the idea that someone should be other than they are, is to practice resisting the impulses to move away and separate ourselves from each other, whether in self-defense or arrogant self-promotion. Can you imagine how peaceful it would feel if we looked to each other for evidence that we are all essentially interconnected and interdependent with each other, rather than separate and on our own? From the former stance, we enable goodwill to flow more easily, which then allows for cooperative transformation.

By definition, divinization is a cooperative experience, as is self-actualization: to actualize, you have to be both inwardly and outwardly focused, which is another beautiful sort of paradox. Enlightenment cannot happen in isolation; it requires not only that we make peace within ourselves, but also that that peace be integrated into the world we live in.

And then, too, we can apply consciousness to our career or work; we can infuse our vocation with meaning and purpose. As the great Buddhist teacher Thich Nhat Hanh so eloquently explains, we can infuse everything we do, even tasks that we might see as mundane like waiting on tables or washing dishes, with the principles of kindness, compassion, and service. The same guiding principles apply, of course, to any profession, from car mechanic to brain surgeon.

In addition, we are challenged to consider our health and well-being from the three key vantage points—body, mind, and spirit, remembering that what is good for one aspect will be good for the other aspects—and with the ultimate goal of recognizing that my good is everyone else's good, and of course, everyone's good is my good.

As such, what we eat affects our health directly, but it also affects our emotions, our spirit, and our totality. And what we choose to eat also affects the world around us in critical ways—our choices can support sustainability, just working conditions, kindness, and other practices that align with our values. In other words, just by what we choose to eat, we can participate in divinization in a very real way.

Let's think about our consumption patterns for a moment: when was the last time you ate something? This is not a rhetorical exercise; before you keep reading, please answer this question for yourself.

Now think about the last time you bought a house.

A car.

Clothing.

If you are like me and like the vast majority of people, you consume more in the form of food than you do everything else combined. Yet, oddly enough, the vast majority of us are deeply disconnected from our food. We don't know where it came from, what went into it, how the workers involved in producing it live, or how the animals were treated or killed if we're eating meat.

So what is "conscious eating" exactly? Basically, conscious eating entails knowing where our food comes from and what goes into making it, and choosing to eat in a way that affirms our integrity and our most basic values. That goes for everything we consume, of course, but with food, it's far more constant (we eat at least three times a day!) and our power to make better choices is far more profound here than with anything else we consume.

I believe that the decisions we make in terms of our food choices are, in a very real way, our deepest connection to our core values and principles. Regarding food preparation, what if we were to ask ourselves: Is the process by which this food has arrived on my plate just? Has compassion been applied? Kindness? Have I done everything I can to not cause suffering, and in fact, have I done anything that might alleviate suffering? After all, if these are the principles—justice, compassion, kindness, and alleviating suffering where I can—that we wish to see in the world, doesn't it make sense that we should question whether or not our sense of integrity is served by what we choose to eat? I believe Socrates would agree.

So the goal of conscious eating is not just to eat food that is delicious and nutritious, though that is certainly key. We also must challenge ourselves to eat foods that are in alignment with our spiritual values, foods that don't involve, as much as possible, exploitation of the earth, workers, or animals.

For me, centering my life around foods that are consciously chosen to support a kinder and more just world has been more life-transforming than any other choice I have ever made. This transition in my life has freed me, at a deep level, and caused me to feel an intensity of satisfaction and power that is far beyond anything I would have expected, vaulting me to a whole new level of well-being, physically, emotionally, and spiritually.

And, in fact, it occurs to me that in addition to the web of relationships formed by eating, and the frequency of our consumption, eating is foundational in another way: we engage in it at multiple times throughout our day, so that for many of us, it adds a rhythm and order to our lives. If our eating is in sync with our values, then our lives have a shot of integrity repeatedly throughout our day.

When I was trying to define my faith, my connection to Spirit, it occurred to me that spiritual principles are geared toward self-realization. And that if I wanted to embody or actualize those principles (so I could become more self-realized), I needed to apply them to the daily ritual of eating. I needed to purchase and eat food with this ever-present question: with this choice, am I supporting kindness or cruelty?

I know that some people will say, "Wait a minute, Kathy, you're talking about food here, not war and peace." Perhaps so, but one of the deep truths that Pythagoras, Tolstoy, Gandhi, Einstein (all vegetarians, incidentally), and so many other extraordinary thinkers grasped and promoted was that if we can't get the little things right, how can we get the big things right? Put another way, if the foundation of our lives (quite literally, eating is how we sustain ourselves for everything else we do) is based in either thoughtlessness or complicity in cruelty or environmental harm, how can the rest of our lives align in a positive manner?

I recall the words of the Apostle Paul in his first letter to the Thessalonians, where he calls on the community to "pray ceaselessly." Since eating is so central to our lives, eating consciously can be the foundation of our conscious life. It can be our constant prayer. As conscious eaters, specifically, we become an active force in the inevitable tide of history—the divinization that Teilhard talked about—that gives us a deeply seated hope and optimism about the future. We become empowered and inspired.

I agree with Socrates that we should lead examined lives, with Gandhi that our lives should be focused on the experiment of truth, and with Teilhard that this truth should focus squarely on advancing not just ourselves but the whole of humanity as global caretakers.

When we realign ourselves in these ways, we will find peace in all aspects of our lives.

Shortly before his death, Teilhard wrote,

> When all is said and done, I can see this: I managed to climb to the point where the Universe became apparent to me as a great rising surge, in which all the work that goes into serious inquiry, all the will to create, all the acceptance of suffering, converge ahead into a single dazzling spearhead—now, at the end of my life, I can stand on the peak I have scaled and continue to look ever more closely into the future, and there, with ever more assurance, see the ascent of God.

The ascent of God—that was Teilhard's way of explaining the positive moral forward march of our species. That is, in my view, what a life dedicated to quantum wellness will attain.

Today's Meditation

I am a bringer of light. I use my life as a vessel through which light can flow and become grounded. Each and every time I act in a way that is conscious and kind, I am actualizing my prayer for peace and healing. I adhere to my principles of compassion and mercy; I alleviate (or don't contribute to) suffering whenever or wherever I am aware of it. I am rising to my highest potential through my daily choices, and thus bringing light into the world.

Day 20:

Awakening

Today I want us to focus on the big picture—of how your food gets to you and what the spiritual effects of that process are. Fair warning: once you do this, there may be no turning back!

I know that several experiences put me over the edge in terms of conscious eating, but I would guess that nothing had the same impact on me as John Robbins's *The Food Revolution* (in its first iteration, it was called *Diet for a New America*). John Robbins, heir to the Baskin-Robbins ice-cream fortune, gave up his inheritance to become a best-selling author of muckraking books in the tradition of Ida Tarbell and Upton Sinclair. In *The Food Revolution*, Robbins goes deeply into the issues of where our food comes from and offers extensive scientific information about the issues that I've only begun to touch on here—the health problems associated with animal products, the ecological issues, the fact that eating meat drives up the price of grains, soy, and corn, contribution to global starvation, and more. As I detailed in *Quantum Wellness*, I had long suspected that there were things I should know about how animals become our food, but for many years I avoided reading the books or watching the videos that revealed the behind-the-scenes truth. I certainly knew that animals were not inanimate objects; I knew that they bled if you pricked them and had personalities and traits that couldn't help but make me realize that they had the same spark of life in them that was in me. But I liked my meat. I liked having grilled steak on the weekends and barbecued chicken with my family. I enjoyed cheesy pizza to no end, and eggs were a mainstay in my diet. There was something so culturally sound about sharing a hamburger with friends, or turkey on Thanksgiving, and I wasn't ready to start tinkering with "the good times."

But as I moved forward in my spiritual life, I began to ask myself, "By choosing to eat this food, am I living according to the principles that are important to me?" Principles like kindness, compassion, mercy, and alleviating of suffering when possible. And, at the very least, I thought, if I wanted to become more awake and aware on my path of spiritual growth, was I looking at things squarely and with open eyes, or was I insisting on keeping my head in the sand? If I were to continue to eat meat, I figured I should know full well the process by which it arrived on my plate.

This was the hardest chapter to write, and I suspect that it will be the most difficult for you to read. But there are certain things that can no longer afford indifference. Even if we choose not to change, it's still important that we understand the world around us, that we understand how our food gets to us.

Anyway, as much as I dreaded it, I started cracking open the books and reading the accounts of what happens in slaughterhouses. I forced myself to sit down and watch the videos provided by animal protection organizations.

I learned that in the United States alone, we now kill almost 10 billion land animals annually, mostly chickens and turkeys, and that almost all these animals (well over 95 percent) are raised in factory farms—or, as the industry calls them, concentrated animal feeding operations, or CAFOs—massive metal sheds in which tens or even hundreds of thousands of animals are crammed, unable to do anything they were designed to do, often so drugged up and genetically altered that they can barely walk, if they can walk at all. Hens have their sensitive beaks seared off, a process that causes intense pain that lasts for more than a month. Pigs have their ears and teeth mutilated without pain relief. All this would be illegal were dogs or cats so horribly abused. And of course, these poor creatures have no idea what is happening to them, and they don't have the power to make it stop.

I also read Gail Eisnitz's book *Slaughterhouse,* and these are some of the passages that haunt me to this day:

> A worker who was angry with his supervisor for pushing him hard said he "could've easily taken a human life and not given it one thought or had one regret for it. . . . It's the same thing with an animal who pisses you off, except it is in the stick pit, you are going to kill it. Only you don't just kill it, you go in hard, push hard, blow the windpipe, make it drown in its own blood. Split its nose. A live hog

would be running around the pit. It would just be looking up at me and I'd be sticking, and I would just take
my knife and—eerk—cut its eye out while it was just sitting there. And this hog would just scream. One time I
took my knife—it's sharp enough—and I sliced off the
end of a hog's nose, just like a piece of bologna. The hog
went crazy for a few seconds. Then it just sat there looking kind of stupid. So I took a handful of salt brine and
ground it into his nose. Now that hog really went nuts,
pushing its nose all over the place. I still had a bunch of
salt left on my hand—I was wearing a rubber glove—and
I stuck the salt right up the hog's ass. The poor hog didn't
know whether to shit or go blind. . . . It's not anything
anyone should be proud of. It happened. It was my way
of taking out frustration."

"Another time, there was a live hog in the pit. It hadn't
done anything wrong, wasn't even running around the pit.
It was just alive. I took a three-foot chunk of pipe—two
inch diameter pipe—and I literally beat that hog to
death. Couldn't have been a two-inch piece of solid
bone left in its head. Basically, if you want to put it in lay-
man's terms, I crushed his skull. It was like I started hit-
ting the hog and I couldn't stop. And when I finally did
stop, I'd expended all this energy and frustration, and I'm
thinking, what in God's sweet name did I do? But I wasn't
the only guy doing this kind of stuff. One guy I work with
actually chases hogs into the scalding tank. And everybody—hog drivers, shacklers, utility men—uses lead
pipes on hogs. Everybody knows it, all of it."

A vet replied, on being asked if he ever saw violations of the Humane Slaughter Act: "Like torching off an animal's leg? A steer was running up the alleyway and got his leg between the boards and he couldn't get it out. They didn't want to lose any time killing cattle, and he was blocking their path, so they just used a blow torch to burn his leg off while he was alive. . . . Cattle dragged and choked, stuff like that. Knocking 'em four, five, ten times. Every now and then when they're stunned they come back to life, and they're up there agonizing. They're supposed to be restunned but sometimes they aren't and they'll go through the skinning process alive. I saw that myself, a bunch of times. I've found them alive clear over to the rump stand. When they're sucking in air and bellowing, their eyes bugging out. Sometimes they fall through the bottom of that restrainer and they're still alive. And the workers have to get them up anyway they can. So, they wrap a chain around it, lift it up, bust something. If it's a leg, they'll break the leg. If it's the head, they'll break the neck. . . . You can hear the bones cracking a lot of times. And that happens in every plant. . . . They're all the same . . . everybody gets so used to it that it doesn't mean anything."

You might say that Eisnitz is describing only the aberrant behavior of a deranged few, and surely these are some pretty extreme scenarios, but the fact is, cruelty and abuse are far more common in our system of industrial meat production than most of us care to think about. And what's "normal" isn't much better. Practices that are "acceptable" and perfectly legal include: beaks, testicles, or horns chopped off without any pain relief; animals trucked through all kinds of extreme weather, their skin frozen against metal trucks; hooves and wings broken in transport; sores festering without relief. The sick or dying are discarded on "dead piles" (the sight of them twitching in pain, eyes wide open, is quite harrowing), dragged to slaughter when they refuse to or can't walk, mothers and babies separated at the moment of birth by force, causing extreme distress.

Just recently I watched a documentary called *45 Days: The Life and Death of a Broiler Chicken*. Again, chickens make up more than 98 percent of all land animals slaughtered in the United States, and they're the most abused of all factory farmed animals. Their lives are miserable from the day they are born until the day they're killed. In this documentary, which you can find easily online by searching by the title, investigators visit the same chicken shed every week for the entire duration of these chickens' lives, forty-five days. At one point in the video, the camera focuses on a little chick on the floor of a "growing shed," among tens of thousands of others. She struggles to get her legs under her, but she can't hold herself up, because like other chickens, drugs and genetic breeding have forced her to swell to an unnaturally large size; her upper body has grown at twice its normal pace, so her legs simply can't sustain the heaviness. This industrious little soul was pulling herself along the feces-covered floor trying as hard as she could to raise herself up, but finally, she gave up and lay with her face in the muck. It's a bit like the "little engine who could," except, for modern chickens, they never make it over the hill.

One thing that strikes me every time I look at a dog, cat,

chicken, pig, or even a fish, is how similar they are to us. They are constructed of the same things (flesh, bone, blood), have the same senses, and are (as Darwin noted) more similar to us than dissimilar from us. The time when this is most profound for me is when I look into an animal's eyes. There is something sacred there, something alive and mysterious and beyond my right to interfere with.

There is a scene that is burned into my consciousness, from a slaughterhouse in Massachusetts; it will never, ever leave me. The video depicts a man coming to drag a pig to her death, and as I looked into the animal's eyes, I saw that same unmistakable spark of life that animates all of us; but more than that, I saw terror. Abject, unmitigated, unmistakable terror. That pig (pigs are incredibly smart and aware) struggled for her life, her eyes darting around madly, looking for relief, for help. And her earsplitting cries were met with utter cold indifference, and even scorn. I wondered what it would feel like to be dragged and shoved to my death like she was, so mechanically and without so much as a nod to the life that was about to be extinguished. I wondered, and continued to wonder, as I pondered my next meal.

Intellectually, I know that other animals feel the same emotions we do. Darwin taught us that, and Richard Dawkins and others continue to hammer the point home. But emotionally, deep in my core, it's the images of animals from videos— of their eyes, registering the horror of what is happening to them, which speaks to me even more deeply, at a more visceral level.

These are, unfortunately, ordinary glimpses into the everyday life of a modern factory farm and slaughterhouse, recognizable to anyone who's ever been in one. This is how animals look—scared and in visible pain—before they arrive at the supermarket in their sterile plastic platters, labels pasted all over them.

For a long time I considered myself to be a spiritual person, even saying grace before my meals, and yet I certainly wasn't *living* in a grace-filled way. As I took in all these grim facts, I knew I had to change.

The words of Ralph Waldo Emerson ring in my ears still: "You have just dined, and, however scrupulously the slaughterhouse is concealed in the graceful distance of miles, there is complicity."

At some point, I had to ask myself, "Am I okay with the spiritual price of this burger or fillet or omelet or ham? Do I really believe there is no other way?" Matthew Scully brings home the point when he writes in his brilliant book *Dominion*: ". . . inside the factory farm, animals. . . received no comforts, no names, no affection, no nothing, only my silent and resolute indifference. . . . All of this not to obey some inexorable force of evolution or biology, not by divine decree, not to meet some unstoppable market demand, not for Everyone—no, all of it done just for me. Each creature bred and born just for me. Confined and isolated just for me. And then in lonely terror packed off to die, just for me. And every time I saw and heard them I would have to remind myself just why I was doing this, to ask if my taste for pork loins or ham or steak or veal was really worth this price, to ask if this was really my choice and there was no other way. . . . Therefore, I want no part in any of it. I do not want this product. And I damn sure don't want someone else doing the confining and beating and killing for me so that I am spared the unpleasantness of it all. The only thing worse than cruelty is delegated cruelty. It is colder than if I were doing it myself. When you eat flesh extracted in this way, as novelist Alice Walker puts it, 'You're just eating misery. You're eating a bitter life. . . .' For me, it comes down to a question of whether I am a man or just a consumer. Whether to reason or just to rationalize. Whether to heed my conscience or my every craving, to assert my free will or just my will. Whether to side with the powerful and comfortable or with the weak, afflicted, and forgotten. Whether, as an economic actor in a free market, I answer to the god of money or to the God of mercy."

As much as I loved my traditions, as much as I liked the taste of animal protein, and as much as I had bought into the idea that we humans need our meat, dairy, and eggs to be strong and healthy, *something deep within me revolted.* For the sake of satiating my desire to eat a little flesh, could I agree to support an industry that so severely deprived a living creature the most basic of mercies? Could I be complicit in denying them their sacred right to live and die without torment? As Scully proposed, "I am betting that in the Book of Life, 'He had mercy on the creatures' is going to count for more than 'He ate well.'" If our food bears the stain of undue cruelty, I wonder how much it can really nourish us. I began to realize that my habits were not really aligned with a higher nature that was trying to emerge in me. The traditions I had cherished might, in fact, go against the eternal laws that I wanted to lean ever further into. After all, is it not part of the process of our becoming spiritually or ethically mature to say "no" to a few cravings or wants as we become aware that certain practices are absolutely abhorrent to our ideals or sense of principle?

And just a word here, lest we cast judgment on the slaughterhouse workers, we might stop and imagine that the people who work in these killing pits are driven fairly mad by the horrors of what they are partaking in, and so become somewhat warped themselves. Or that some sort of mechanism kicks in and they simply stop feeling, because to truly feel it would mean suffering at the dark gravity of what they are doing. They say as much in interviews; they are also victims.

There is a nearly 100 percent turnover in slaughterhouses each year. Laborers who need the work can't even bear to stay there. Says *New York Times* writer Charlie LeDuff: "Slaughtering . . . is repetitive, brutish work. . . . Five thousand quit and five thousand are hired every year. You hear people say, 'they don't kill pigs in the plant, they kill people.'" One has to wonder at the cost to our humanity to slaughter 10 billion land animals each year in the United States alone—*10 billion* live, feeling creatures who experience extreme fear and pain.

As you hang in through the final days of your cleanse, think about the foods you are now choosing to put on your plate, and how good it feels to know that, if even just for now, you are not participating in the barbarism of the factory farming of animals. Think of these words of Mahatma Gandhi and realize that you can actually move forward and participate in the bettering of yourself and the world:

> The world of tomorrow will be, must be, a society based on non-violence. . . . It may seem a distant goal, an im-

practical Utopia. But it is not in the least unobtainable, since it can be worked for here and now. An individual can adopt the way of life of the future—the nonviolent way—without having to wait for others to do so. And if an individual can do it, cannot whole groups of individuals? Whole nations?

Change happens within individuals first, and then it ripples out and gains momentum. I hope the cleanse is allowing you the time to contemplate your place in the whole.

Consider, then, this passage from Genesis: "And God said, 'Behold, I have given you every herb bearing seed, which is upon the face of all the earth, and every tree, in which is the fruit of a tree yielding fruit; to you it shall be for meat.'" The fact is, we have been provided for, without needing to kill an animal. We can get everything we need—protein, iron, good taste, etc.—without compromising our spiritual integrity.

Today's Meditation

The mantra of the day seems to have become clear: *I awaken.* I am no longer asleep. What is good for my body is good for my soul. I can take a huge leap as I move along the continuum of consciousness by staying alert and adhering to the great wisdom passed down through the ages that advises us to be loving, merciful, and compassionate. I am no longer willing to be greedy, gluttonous, or ignorant. Eating with spiritual integrity is of the utmost importance.

Day 21:

The Leap

THIS IS IT! YOUR FINAL DAY OF THE CLEANSE.

I am consistently humbled by all the people who tell me they completed this cleanse and feel better for it. I designed it for my own edification and certainly didn't expect to be putting it into a book. I consider it the greatest possible gift that you've just given over twenty-one days of your life to this cleanse, and my deepest hope is that you've found the journey to be valuable and rewarding.

The way I see it is this: you have accomplished something magnificent. You have challenged yourself to rethink the way you eat, drink, consume, and relate—the very fundamentals of life. And you've not only thought about it, but you have acted on it. By abstaining from the Big Five for twenty-one days, you have pulled yourself up and out of old habits and delivered yourself to a new peak of wellness. This is not easy stuff, for habits come about because they are comfortable— you know who you are and how you fit in when you maintain old familiar behaviors and dynamics. You know how you will feel, and what to expect.

It's human nature to maintain the status quo; by remaining locked into old ways, we can feel like we are in control; we know what's coming around the bend, and there won't be any great surprises. By shifting gears the way you have, you lifted yourself up and into unknown territory. Of course you knew it would be a healthy move for you (that's why you did it) but you overcame your resistance to change. And that's nothing to take lightly.

That said, though, it's also in our inherent nature to grow and expand, and new vistas are surprisingly wonderful. Once you start thinking deeply about things, it's nearly impossible to ignore an almost urgent impulse to push forward, past the constraints of thinking just of yourself and into a more unified vision of a compassionate and inclusive world. The subtle whispers of your soul that guided you to explore where a cleanse could take you have likely delivered you right into the heart of a personal, and then cultural, revolution.

As you continue to put into practice a self-improvement plan—engaging in self-inquiry and working at overcoming baser instincts—you will yield improvements not only for yourself, but for the larger society. You will join the wave of pioneers, taking bold steps into a yet to be formed brighter future. This is how we make our way to the next stage of human achievement and evolution: one step at a time, one illumination at a time.

Remember how we talked about the power of small things to change your entire mood? That power applies even more profoundly to the power of small changes in your being to influence bigger and growing changes in society. This concept is actually the base of positive social change. For example, just one woman—Rosa Parks—refused to sit in the back of the bus, and a civil rights revolution was sparked.

In these past twenty-one days, you have had the experience of:

- **Eating in a way that energizes your body and prevents disease.**
- **Being free from habits that drained your life force.**
- **Instilling new practices—meditation, visualization, self-inquiry, spiritual practice—that bring forth and sustain health and happiness.**
- **Making conscious choices so that you align yourself with your core values of kindness, compassion, and right living.**

You've essentially taken a quantum leap from your old ways of being and delivered yourself into an altogether higher state. You've worked on lots of things at once, which is actually how "momentous change" happens. By tweaking and upgrading the various aspects of body, mind, and spirit simultaneously, we stoke the fire of self-transcendence from every direction, pushing forward a serious momentum of change. Let this be the new upward mobility—the evolutionary urge to go beyond ourselves, to transcend where we currently reside, and to answer the call for deep transformation.

This is the spiritual priority a cleanse like this calls forth: to consciously and continuously pursue our own evolution. As we read and think deeply about the suffering of animals and workers and the degradation of the planet that results from our old ways of eating, we realize that we are tasked with cultivating new traditions—in our homes and in our communities—that bring forth a worldview that is inclusive and kind rather than narcissistic and gluttonous. We are moving away from a culture of "me first," which strove to gratify immediate hungers, and into a more mindful culture of integration and conscious consumption. We are healing ourselves so that we can, in turn, be the healers this world so sorely needs.

Yes, you may now introduce back into your diet any of the Big Five. Of course I urge you to think carefully about how to do this, so you don't give your body a shock by loading it with heavy stressors all at once.

The first thing to reintroduce (if you want) should be gluten. See how your body responds. Give it a few days and see how your gut feels, how your energy and mood are affected. If you aren't having any problems after a few days, you can count yourself among the lucky ones who don't have gluten sensitivities. Go slowly with the alcohol, please. Now that your body has detoxed a bit from its effects, you will probably have a more intense reaction to it than you're used to, and the sugar load on top of the alcohol will probably give you more of a buzz than you bargained for. And stay away from processed sugar, using healthy substitutes instead. You've been experiencing the wonderful benefits of balanced blood sugar. Why compromise that now?

What to say about caffeine? I still enjoy it occasionally, and if you've really missed it, go ahead and have some. But maybe now you'll find you don't need or can't even tolerate as much of it to get you going. Maybe a cup of tea or half-strength coffee will do the trick in the morning. Try it and see.

Last but certainly not least, I am hoping you've decided to continue to eat a plant-based diet. As we've seen, there are just too many reasons not to eat animal protein—for our own health, the environment, the global poor, and of course for the animals. You've experienced it yourself. We don't need animal protein. And *everyone* and *everything* benefits from your move to a plant-based diet.

As you conclude your cleanse, ask yourself these questions:

- What have I learned by doing this cleanse?
- What are the material or practical lessons?
- What are the inner lessons?
- How can I keep pushing this upward thrust of growth?
- What do I need to do in order to make this peak experience a permanent upgrade?

Let the answers to these questions settle into and guide your daily practices. Reflect on them as you continue to overcome all your previous defenses and awaken new convictions. This is a heroic (and sometimes arduous!) endeavor you've undertaken, to construct new pillars of wellness. Keep your eye on the horizon as you continue to build, for you are helping to create the new structures upon which we will hoist ourselves up and into a superior existence.

Perhaps you didn't think you could do it. Maybe you had a few slips. But now you know just how powerful you are. Now you know that you are the healer who can heal yourself and extend that healing out into the world. *May you be well and thrive in every respect, and may you use this foundation of power to help move us all forward.*

Recipes

HERE'S THE FUN PART—THE FOOD! THE FOLLOWING ARE some delicious recipes by my dear friend Tal Ronnen and his associate, Lex Townes. Tal is a chef who has made it his mission to create food that is completely plant-based, incredibly tasty, and nutritious. He is a genius in the kitchen, and the recipes bear the mark of his commitment to showing people how to eat consciously (and still be fulfilled and satisfied!). I gave Tal the challenge of not only coming up with incredibly sumptuous vegan meals, but also to do them without sugar or gluten. These are, of course, just some of the delicious dishes you can eat while on the cleanse. Try them, change them up, and add ingredients that are in season where you live. Please enjoy!

BREAKFASTS

CHERRY COCONUT BREAKFAST BARS

½ cup vegan butter

½ cup agave nectar

2¼ cups steel-cut oats (uncooked)

1 cup shredded coconut

1 tsp. baking powder

3 Tbsp. sesame seeds

½ cup pitted prunes, chopped

½ cup dried apricots, chopped

½ cup dried cherries

1 banana, smashed well against the side of a bowl

Egg replacer equivalent to 2 eggs (use Ener-G
    brand), prepared according to the instructions
    on the box

Preheat the oven to 350°F.

Put the vegan butter and agave in a small pan over medium heat and stir until melted.

In a large bowl, mix the oats, coconut, baking powder, and sesame seeds. Add the prunes, apricots, and cherries and mix well.

Gently fold in the prepared egg replacer.

Add the agave mixture and banana and mix. Pour into a square baking pan.

Bake for 25 minutes, or until cooked through. Let cool, remove from the pan, and cut into rectangular bars.

Makes 9 bars.

Tofu Scramble Breakfast Sandwich with Tempeh Bacon and Oven Roasted Tomatoes

1 (16-oz.) container firm water-packed tofu, drained
    and pressed
2 tsp. olive oil, plus more for brushing the tomatoes
1 small onion, sliced
2 oz. sliced shiitake mushrooms
3 Tbsp. nutritional yeast flakes
½ tsp. onion powder
1 tsp. turmeric
1 garlic clove, minced
2 Tbsp. wheat-free soy sauce
2 medium tomatoes
Salt and pepper to taste
8 slices smoked tempeh bacon
8 slices gluten-free bread

Place the tofu between two paper towels and press out the water.

Heat the olive oil in a sauté pan and sauté the onion and mushrooms for 3 minutes. Crumble the tofu into the pan and add the nutritional yeast, onion powder, turmeric, garlic, and soy sauce. Cook for about 7 minutes, stirring occasionally.

Cut the tomatoes into 1-inch-thick slices, coat with olive oil, season with salt and pepper, and roast in the oven at 350°F for 15 minutes, flipping halfway through the cooking time.

Crisp the "bacon" in a pan. Place two strips on four slices of wheat-free bread and top with a tomato slice and some of the tofu scramble mixture.

Makes 4 sandwiches.

TOFU SCRAMBLE

2–3 Tbsp. extra-virgin olive oil

1 sweet onion, cut into chunks

5 garlic cloves, minced

2 Tbsp. nutritional yeast

½ tsp. ground ginger

½ tsp. chili powder

½ yellow or green bell pepper, seeded and chopped

1 cup sliced mushrooms

4 tomatoes, chopped

1 lb. firm tofu, drained well and cut into bite-size
   pieces

Tamari to taste

Freshly ground pepper to taste

Fresh snipped chives to taste

Heat the olive oil over medium heat in a large skillet and sauté the onion for 5 minutes, until softened.

Add the garlic, nutritional yeast, and spices, stir, and cook for 1 minute. Add the pepper and mushrooms, stir-frying until tender and crisp.

Add the tomatoes and chopped tofu. Gently stir-fry for 3 to 4 minutes. Sprinkle with the tamari sauce and season with fresh pepper and chives.

Makes 4 servings.

Breakfast Cookies
(by Todd Lindeberg)

2 cups pomegranate juice

1 cup steel-cut oats

1 cup raw almonds

1 cup raw pumpkin seeds

1 cup goji berries

1 cup mashed banana

½ cup freshly ground peanut butter

¼ cup vegan butter (try Earth Balance brand)

Bring the pomegranate juice to a boil in a saucepan and add the steel-cut oats.

Cook until just starts to boil, then remove from the heat immediately, cover, and allow to absorb and cool.

Place the rest of the ingredients in a food processor and blend to mix.

When the oats are cool, mix with the rest of the ingredients to form a wet cookie dough.

Place the dough in the middle of a 2-foot-long piece of plastic wrap and roll into a log shape. Tie both ends, ensuring that the cookie dough is airtight.

Freeze until needed.

When ready to use, defrost till just soft enough to cut into ½-inch slices.

Preheat the oven to 400°F.

Bake on parchment paper for 10 minutes, then turn off the oven and continue to dehydrate until cool.

Makes 24 cookies.

*Note: I like to reheat them every morning and pour my daily dose of 2 Tbsp. flax oil on top!

LUNCHES

BLACK BEAN VEGGIE BURGERS

2–4 Tbsp. olive oil

½ cup diced red onion

½ cup diced green bell pepper

1 clove garlic, minced

1 jalapeño, minced

2 cups cooked black beans, drained but not rinsed

½ cup corn kernels

½ cup bread crumbs made from gluten-free bread*

½ tsp. cumin

2 Tbsp. chopped cilantro

1 tsp. salt

½ cup spelt flour

In a saucepan over medium heat, in 1 tablespoon of the olive oil, sauté the onion, bell pepper, garlic, and jalapeño for 4 to 5 minutes. Remove from heat and set aside.

In a mixing bowl, mash the black beans, then add the sautéed vegetables, corn, and bread crumbs, and mix well. Season with cumin, cilantro, and salt, and mix again.

Shape into six patties, then coat each in spelt flour.

Place a pan over medium-high heat and add the remaining tablespoon of oil. Cook each patty for about 5 minutes on each side, or until lightly browned, adding more oil to the pan as needed.

*Note: To make gluten-free bread crumbs, break a loaf of gluten-free bread into pieces and process in a food processor until reduced to crumbs. Spread the bread crumbs on a cookie sheet and bake at 300°F for 10 minutes, or until toasted.

Makes 6 small patties.

Tempeh Tuna Salad

4 slices fresh ginger (slice a whole root thinly across
   the width; no need to peel)
2¼ cups vegetable broth
1 tsp. sea salt
½ orange
1 (8 oz.) package tempeh
Juice of 1 lemon
3 Tbsp. tamari
1 clove garlic, minced
½ cup finely minced red onion
1 Tbsp. dry seaweed flakes
3 ribs celery, finely chopped
¾ cup chopped kosher pickles
¼ cup vegan mayonnaise (try Vegenaise brand)

Place the ginger, vegetable broth, and sea salt in a sauce pan.

Squeeze the juice from the orange half into the pot and then add the spent half to the pot.

Place the entire uncut tempeh block into the pot, bring to a simmer, and cook on low heat for 45 minutes to 1 hour, or until the tempeh block is softened but not falling apart.

Allow the tempeh to cool in the liquid.

Remove the tempeh from the liquid and grate on the large side of a box grater to create a coarse tempeh mixture.

In a separate bowl, combine all the remaining ingredients and mix well.

Add to the tempeh and stir well to combine.

Optional: Serve over mixed greens and garnish with thinly sliced scallions.

Makes approximately 5 servings.

BAKED EGGPLANT, SQUASH, AND AMARANTH WRAPS

1 medium eggplant, sliced lengthwise into long,
    thin slices
1 zucchini squash, sliced lengthwise into long, thin
    slices
1 yellow squash, sliced lengthwise into long, thin
    slices
2 Tbsp. olive oil
Sprinkling of salt and black pepper

Place the vegetable slices in a single layer on baking sheets.

Brush with the oil, coating both sides well.

Sprinkle salt and pepper lightly over both sides.

Bake at 425°F for 10 to 15 minutes, or until softened but not mushy.

For the amaranth:
2¼ cups water
1 cup whole amaranth seeds

1 bay leaf
2 sprigs fresh thyme
2 tsp. salt
3 Tbsp. olive oil
Juice of 1 lemon
¼ cup chopped parsley
1½ tsp. salt
Cracked black pepper, to taste

Bring the water to a simmer and add the amaranth, bay leaf, thyme sprigs, and salt.

Cook, covered, for 20 minutes, or until the grain is softened and the water has been absorbed (adding more water, if necessary, to cook fully).

Stir in the remaining ingredients and reserve. Remove thyme sprigs and bay leaf.

To assemble:
5 gluten-free tortillas (try Don Pancho brand)
3 Tbsp. vegan mayonnaise (try Vegenaise)
1 cup baby spinach
1 red onion, sliced thinly
Cooked amaranth
Cooked eggplant and squashes, p. 178

Place the tortillas on a cookie sheet and warm briefly in a 350°F oven for 1 to 2 minutes. (Or open the package of tortillas and microwave for about 45 seconds.)

Lay each tortilla down flat. Slather generously with the vegan mayonnaise.

Next, lay leaves of spinach on the tortillas, followed by slices of red onion, and then top with about ⅓ of the cooked amaranth and slices of the cooked eggplant and squashes.

Place ingredients in the middle of the tortilla, leaving 2 inches of outside free of ingredients.

Folding like an envelope, bring bottom flap up and then fold in both sides. Roll over one time to complete envelope effect.

Cut in half on angle from corner to corner.

Makes 5 wraps.

MIDDLE EASTERN SWEET-POTATO SALAD ON ROMAINE LEAVES WITH WARM CHIPOTLE TOFU BATONS

For the salad:
    5 Tbsp. olive oil
    ½ onion, diced
    1½ lb. sweet potatoes, peeled and cubed
    Water
    1 tsp. grated fresh ginger
    1 tsp. cumin
    1 tsp. paprika
    1½ tsp. salt
    ¼ cup pitted green olives, chopped
    Juice of ½ lemon
    3 Tbsp. chopped parsley
    4 or 5 whole romaine leaves, washed and dried

In a medium saucepan, heat 2 Tbsp. of the oil over medium heat and sauté the onion until translucent.

Add the sweet potatoes and just enough water to cover.

Add the ginger, cumin, paprika, salt, and remaining oil.

Simmer over medium heat until the potatoes are tender and the sauce has reduced, about 15 to 20 minutes.

Remove from the heat and toss with the olives, lemon juice, and parsley.

Place an even amount of the potato salad on each romaine leaf. Set aside.

For the tofu:

> 1 lb. extra-firm tofu, drained
> 2 tsp. agave nectar
> 2 Tbsp. olive oil
> ½ tsp. chipotle in adobo sauce, minced to form a paste
> ½ tsp. salt

Slice the drained tofu through the length to form ½-inch-thick slabs.

Place between two clean towels and gently press to remove excess water.

Cut the slabs across the width to make long, rectangular logs of about ½ inch in cross-section.

Combine the remaining ingredients well in a mixing bowl.

Add the tofu and gently toss to coat well.

Place the tofu pieces on a cookie sheet and position under an open-flame oven broiler, as close to the flame as possible.

Broil for about 10 to 12 minutes, turning to expose each side to the flame, or until well browned and most of the liquid is evaporated.

Remove from the cookie sheet and serve warm over the salad, dividing among salad plates.

Makes 4 or 5 servings.

CURRY TEMPEH SALAD WITH FLAX CRACKERS

8 Tbsp. wheat-free tamari

8 slices fresh ginger

2 one-inch pieces kombu (sea vegetable found in most health food stores)

¼ tsp. sea salt

2 garlic cloves, sliced

6 cups water

1 package tempeh

¾ cup vegan mayonnaise (try Vegenaise)

4 tsp. curry powder

1 Tbsp. fresh lime juice

1 tsp. agave nectar

½ tsp. ground ginger

½ tsp. salt

¼ tsp. black pepper

1 medium red onion, small dice

1 cup red seedless grapes, halved

½ cup coarsely chopped salted roasted cashews

In a large pot, combine the tamari, ginger, kombu, sea salt, sliced garlic, and water. Add the tempeh and let simmer for 1 hour.

Cool the tempeh, pat dry, and crumble into a bowl. Add the rest of the ingredients and mix well.

Makes 4 servings.

CREAMY ITALIAN WHITE-BEAN SOUP

1 lb. dried cannellini beans
6–8 cups cold water
2 Tbsp. olive oil
1 large onion, chopped
3 garlic cloves, crushed
1 tsp. fresh thyme
1 tsp. fresh oregano
2 bay leaves
8 cups faux-chicken or vegetable stock (Pacific
    Natural is a gluten-free, low-sodium option)
1 cup diced tomato
¼ cup chopped fresh basil
Juice of ½ lemon
Salt and pepper, to taste

Place the beans in a large pot and cover with water. Let soak overnight and then drain and set aside.

Heat the olive oil in a large pot over medium heat. Add the onion and cook for 5 minutes. Add the garlic and cook for another minute. Add the beans, thyme, oregano, and bay leaves. Stir in the stock and bring to a boil. Lower the heat, cover the pot, and allow to gently simmer for 2 hours, or until the beans are tender.

Allow to cool slightly and then remove the bay leaves. Purée half the soup in a food processor or blender, then return to the pot.

Add the diced tomato, basil, and lemon juice and season with salt and pepper.

Makes 8 servings.

EDAMAME SOBA SALAD WITH MISO VINAIGRETTE

For the vinaigrette:
2 Tbsp. agave nectar
1 Tbsp. rice vinegar
1 Tbsp. yellow miso
½ Tbsp. grated fresh ginger
1 clove minced garlic
½ cup olive oil

In a bowl, mix the agave nectar, vinegar, miso, ginger, and garlic. Slowly add the olive oil while still stirring. Season with salt and pepper and then set aside.

For the noodles:
1 cup frozen shelled edamame
8 to 9 oz. thin rice noodles
2 Tbsp. vegetable oil
2 Tbsp. finely chopped fresh ginger
2 garlic cloves, chopped

6 scallions, thinly sliced on an angle
1 Tbsp. toasted sesame seeds

Blanch the edamame in a pasta pot of boiling salted water for 4 to 5 minutes. Remove the edamame from the boiling water and cook the pasta until the noodles are tender, following package directions. Drain and set aside.

Heat the oil in a skillet over medium-high heat, then sauté the ginger and garlic for about 30 seconds. Add the scallions and cook for an additional 1 to 2 minutes.

In a large bowl, toss the noodles and edamame with the vinaigrette, ginger, garlic, and scallions. Top with the sesame seeds and serve warm.

Makes 4 servings.

BAKED TOFU OVER RED LENTIL AND SWEET ONION STEW WITH MICRO GREENS

For the tofu:
1 lb. firm tofu
¼ cup vegetable stock (Pacific Natural is a gluten-free, low-sodium option)
3 Tbsp. wheat-free tamari
2 tsp. toasted-sesame oil
2 garlic cloves, minced
1 tsp. minced ginger
½ tsp. black pepper

Wrap the block of tofu in a clean, lint-free towel and place in a colander in the sink. Put a plate and a heavy can or other weight on top of the towel-covered tofu for 30 minutes to drain the water.

Preheat the oven to 350°F.

Remove the tofu from the towel and cut into ½-inch slices. Lightly oil a 9-by-13-inch pan, place the tofu slices in the pan in a single layer, and set aside.

In a small bowl, whisk together the remaining ingredients and pour the mixture over the tofu slices.

Bake for 15 minutes. Remove the pan from the oven, carefully turn the tofu, and bake for 10 to 15 minutes longer, or until all the liquid has been absorbed.

For the lentils:

2 cups dry red (or any color) lentils

2 Tbsp. vegetable oil

1 medium carrot, finely diced

1 large sweet onion (Vidalia, Walla-Walla, Texas
        sweet, Maui sweet, or any sweet onion
        will work), cut into thin, 2-inch-long slices

2 garlic cloves, chopped

3 cups vegetable stock (Pacific Natural is a gluten-
        free, low-sodium option)

½ cup diced tomatoes

1 bay leaf

2 tsp. chopped fresh tarragon

1 Tbsp. vegan butter (try Earth Balance brand)

Salt and freshly cracked black pepper to taste

1 cup micro greens (any kind will work; sunflower
        or radish sprouts may be substituted)

Rinse the lentils well in a strainer under cold running water to remove any dirt.

Heat the oil in a stock pot and add the carrot and onion.

Cook on medium heat for 10 to 12 minutes, or until the onions begin to brown and the carrots are softened.

Add the garlic and cook for an additional minute.

Place the stock, tomatoes, bay leaf, and lentils in the pot, bring to a simmer. Cook for 15 to 20 minutes, or until the lentils have softened and most of the liquid is absorbed.

Stir in the tarragon and vegan butter and season with salt and cracked black pepper.

Place the stew in bowls, top with the baked tofu, and place a small pile of micro greens on top to garnish.

Makes 8 or 9 servings.

HOMEMADE CAESAR DRESSING

16 oz. soft tofu, drained
½ cup lemon juice
6 garlic cloves, crushed
4 Tbsp. tahini
4 Tbsp. capers
1 tsp. Dijon mustard
Salt and pepper to taste
1 cup extra-virgin olive oil
2 Tbsp. fresh parsley

In a blender, combine the tofu, lemon juice, garlic cloves, tahini, capers, Dijon mustard, salt and pepper.

While blending, slowly add the olive oil and process until the mixture is smooth. Add the parsley and pulse a few times.

Makes about 3½ cups. This dressing will keep in the refrigerator for 4 to 5 days.

SCAMPI-STYLE TOFU WRAP

4 Tbsp. olive oil

1 tsp. red-pepper flakes

4 garlic cloves, crushed

1 pound extra-firm tofu, cut into ½-inch cubes

1½ tsp. vegan steak seasoning (try Montreal Steak
     Seasoning by McCormick)

2 hearts romaine lettuce, chopped

3 Tbsp. capers

Juice and zest of 1 lemon

Salt and pepper to taste

4 spinach tortilla wraps, 9- or 10-inch diameter

Heat a large sauté pan over medium-high heat.

Add 2 Tbsp. of the olive oil, the red-pepper flakes, and the garlic. Add the tofu and the steak seasoning. Cook for 6 to 8 minutes, stirring frequently, until the tofu is browned. Transfer to a plate and let cool.

Place the lettuce in a large bowl. Add the cooled tofu, the capers, and the lemon juice and zest. Toss with the remaining oil and season with the salt and pepper.

Heat the tortillas briefly to soften. Fill with the tofu mixture and wrap like a burrito, folding the ends to enclose the filling.

Makes 4 servings.

BASMATI AND BLACK-EYED PEA PILAF WITH HERB-ROASTED VEGETABLES

For the pilaf:
4 Tbsp. vegetable oil
1 medium onion, diced
1 medium red or yellow pepper, diced
1 medium carrot, diced
2 cloves garlic, chopped
1½ cups basmati rice, rinsed well
3 cups vegetable stock (Pacific Natural is a gluten-free, low-sodium option)
3 sprigs fresh thyme
1 bay leaf
3 (15-oz.) cans cooked black-eyed peas, drained well
2 Tbsp. vegan butter (try Earth Balance brand)
Salt and black pepper to taste

Heat the oil in a sauté pan and sweat the onion, pepper, and carrot in the oil for 3 minutes, or until tender.

Add the garlic and cook for 1 minute longer.

Add the rice, stock, thyme, and bay leaf. Bring to a simmer, and cook, covered, for 30 to 45 minutes, or until the rice has softened and most of the liquid is absorbed.

Place the cooked black-eyed peas in a separate pot with the vegan butter and heat through.

Add the cooked rice to the beans, season with salt and pepper, and stir well to combine.

For the vegetables:
½ cup olive oil
3 garlic cloves, minced
2 tsp. chopped fresh tarragon
1½ tsp. chopped fresh thyme
1 tsp. chopped fresh rosemary
4 large portobello mushroom caps, stems removed
1 pint cherry or teardrop tomatoes, cut into
    halves
1 bunch very thin asparagus, hard ends cut off and
    discarded
1 red pepper, seeded and cut into quarters
1 yellow pepper, seeded and cut into quarters
Salt and freshly cracked black pepper to taste

In a small bowl, mix together the oil, garlic, and herbs and set aside.

Remove the black gills from the underside of the mushroom caps by running a spoon against the underside, gently detaching the gills without cutting into the flesh of the mushrooms.

Place the mushrooms, tomato halves, asparagus, and pepper quarters on cookie sheets in one layer, brush liberally with the herbed oil, and season lightly with salt and pepper. (Note: It's important to pack the vegetables loosely on the cookie sheets.)

Roast the vegetables in a preheated 450°F oven for 12 to 15 minutes, or until softened.

Slice the portobello caps on a diagonal to form long, elegant slices and distribute the vegetables evenly over 5 to 6 dishes of the rice pilaf.

Makes 5 to 6 servings

ARUGULA WITH FRESH CITRUS, HEIRLOOM TOMATOES, SHAVED SWEET ONION, AND SESAME-CRUSTED TOFU STEAKS

For the dressing:
2 oranges
1 lemon
1 lime
1 cup orange juice
½ cup white-wine vinegar
1 medium shallot, chopped
2 sprigs fresh thyme
1½ tsp. Dijon mustard
½ cup extra virgin olive oil
Cracked pepper and sea salt, to taste

Zest about 1 Tbsp. of the orange peel and 1 tsp. each of the lemon and lime peel by rasping the fruit on the fine side of a grater, being careful to stop before reaching the bitter white pith.

Cut the orange, lemon, and lime in half and then juice all into a small saucepot.

Add the vinegar, shallot, and thyme to the pan and simmer for 10 minutes, or until syrupy.

Remove from the heat and strain the entire mixture into a food processor.

Add the mustard and slowly drizzle in the olive oil to create a creamy dressing. (*Note:* This may also be done by hand in a bowl by slowly whisking the oil into the ingredients.)

Season with cracked pepper and salt.

For the tofu steaks:

1½ lb. extra-firm tofu, drained well (try White Wave brand)

1 cup brown-rice flour

1 cup unsweetened soy milk

½ tsp. salt

½ tsp. black pepper

1½ cups yellow cornmeal

4 Tbsp. white sesame seeds

4 Tbsp. black sesame seeds

¼ cup canola oil

2 tsp. salt

1 tsp. pepper

Slice the tofu across the width of the block into rectangles of about ½-inch thickness, creating about 10 to 12 slices.

Place the rice flour in a bowl.

Place the soy milk, ½ tsp. salt, and ½ tsp. pepper in a small bowl or pan for dredging the tofu.

Mix the cornmeal, sesame seeds, and 2 tsp. salt and 1 tsp. pepper in a separate bowl.

Coat each tofu slice with the flour and then with the soy milk to moisten.

Place each tofu slice into the cornmeal mixture and gently pat on each side to evenly adhere the crust to the slices.

Heat the oil in a large skillet. (To test for readiness, place a small amount of breading in the oil—when it immediately begins cooking, the oil is ready.)

With tongs, carefully place the tofu slices in the oil and sear on medium-high heat for 3 minutes on each side, or until well browned and heated through. It may be necessary to do this in batches; do not overload the pan.

Drain the tofu on paper towels.

To assemble:
1½ cups organic arugula, washed
Reserved citrus segments
Heirloom tomatoes (1 red and 1 green, or whatever
    looks best at the market), seeded and sliced
    into thin wedges
¼ cup shaved sweet onion (Vidalia, Walla-Walla,
    Maui, or Peruvian sweet; Texas sweets are in
    right now)
Prepared dressing
Warm tofu steaks

Toss the greens, reserved citrus segments, tomatoes, and onions with enough dressing to moisten. Arrange evenly on 5 plates and top with the warm tofu steaks.

Makes 5 entrée salads.

CURRY TEMPEH AND CAULIFLOWER WITH SWEET PEAS OVER JASMINE RICE

For the tempeh:
1½ lb. tempeh (about 3 blocks)
4 cups vegetable stock (Pacific Natural is a gluten-
    free, low-sodium option)
1½ tsp. curry powder
½ tsp. salt

Cut across the width of the tempeh blocks in a diagonal fashion to create slices about 2 inches wide by ½ inch thick.

Place the tempeh slices and all the other ingredients in a flat-bottomed pan that's big enough to hold the tempeh in one layer.

Bring to a simmer and cook for 20 to 25 minutes, or until the tempeh has softened but is not falling apart.

Reserve in the warm liquid.

For the rice:
2 cups jasmine rice
3 cups vegetable stock (Pacific Natural is a gluten-
    free, low-sodium option)

1 bay leaf
1½ tsp. salt

Combine all the ingredients in a stockpot, bring to a simmer, and cook for 30 minutes, or until all the liquid is absorbed and the rice is softened.

Stir once and set aside.

For the curry:
1 head cauliflower
1 medium russet potato, peeled and cut into ½-inch
    dice
⅓ cup vegetable oil
2 medium shallots, sliced
3 Tbsp. curry powder
1 tsp. ground ginger
½ tsp. ground cardamom
1 clove garlic, chopped
2⅓ cups green peas, thawed
2 cups coconut milk
2 tsp. salt

Remove the florets from the cauliflower stem to create small pieces.

Place in simmering water for 3 minutes, or until just beginning to soften.

Plunge the florets into ice water to cool completely.

Cook the potatoes in simmering water for 3 to 4 minutes until just tender. Drain and set aside.

Heat the oil in a sauté pan and cook the shallots over medium-high heat for 5 minutes, or until softened.

Add the the curry, ginger, and cardamom, and cook for 3 minutes to release the spices' aromas.

Add the garlic and cook for an additional minute. Add the cauliflower and cook for about 1 minute, stirring to coat with the spices and oil.

Add the par-cooked potatoes, peas, coconut milk, and salt and cook for 5 minutes, or until heated through. The cooked potatoes will slightly thicken the sauce.

Serve over the hot rice.

Discard the tempeh poaching liquid and place the warm tempeh on top of the dish and serve.

Makes 5 to 6 servings.

SPICY GRILLED TEMPEH AND SQUASH OVER EGYPTIAN SAUTÉED FAVA BEANS WITH ROASTED PEPPER SAUCE

For the sauce:
⅔ cup jarred roasted red peppers, drained well
Juice of ½ lemon
½ tsp. salt
¼ tsp. pepper
1 cup vegan mayonnaise (try Vegenaise)
2 Tbsp. extra-virgin olive oil

Place all the ingredients except the olive oil in a food processor and blend until smooth.

With the machine running, drizzle in the olive oil to form a creamy sauce.

For the Tempeh:
1 lb. tempeh
½ cup olive oil
½ cup gluten-free tamari
¼ cup plus 1 Tbsp. lime juice
3 cloves garlic, minced
2 Tbsp. chipotle in adobo, minced very finely into
    a paste
1 Tbsp. salt
2 tsp. ground coriander
1 tsp. ground cumin

Slice the tempeh across the width at an angle to create ¼-inch-thick flat slices.

Combine all the other ingredients in a bowl and mix well.

Gently toss the tempeh slices in the marinade, place in a flat dish, cover, and let sit in the refrigerator for 2 hours or overnight.

Remove the slices from the marinade and grill for 2 to 3 minutes on each side, or until well marked by the grill and cooked completely through.

For the squash:
2 small zucchini, cut in half lengthwise and seeded
2 small yellow squash, cut in half lengthwise and
    seeded

3 Tbsp. olive oil
Salt and pepper to taste

Cut each zucchini and squash half into 3 pieces on an angle.
   Coat each with olive oil.
   Sprinkle liberally with salt and pepper.
   Grill with the tempeh for about 3 minutes per side.

For the fava beans:
2 Tbsp. olive oil
2 shallots, finely diced
1 garlic clove, minced
1 large tomato, seeds removed and diced
1 (15-oz.) can fava beans, drained and rinsed
1 tsp. ground cumin
1 tsp. crushed red pepper
½ tsp. smoked paprika (regular paprika may be
   substituted)
Salt and pepper to taste
¼ cup chopped fresh parsley
3 Tbsp. lemon juice

Heat the olive oil in a medium saucepan and sauté the shallots for 3 minutes.
   Add the garlic and tomato and cook for 4 more minutes.
   Add the beans, cumin, red pepper, paprika, salt, and pepper, and simmer on medium heat for 10 minutes.
   Add the fresh parsley and lemon juice and simmer for 2 more minutes.

Distribute the beans evenly among 5 to 6 plates.

Place about 2 oz. of the sauce around the outside of the beans and top with the grilled tempeh and squash.

Makes 5 to 6 servings.

ROASTED GARLIC, BEANS, AND GREENS WITH SUN-DRIED TOMATO RISOTTO AND PINE NUTS

For the greens:
Head of garlic
6 Tbsp. olive oil (3 for roasting the garlic)
2 heads escarole, roughly chopped
1 Tbsp. chopped fresh parsley
1 Tbsp. chopped basil
Salt and pepper to taste
¼ tsp. crushed red pepper flakes
2 (16-oz.) cans cannellini beans, undrained

Preheat the oven to 350°F.

Cut the tips off the head of garlic, exposing the cloves, and drizzle with half of the olive oil. Wrap in foil and bake for 25 minutes.

In a sauté pan, heat the remaining 3 tablespoons of olive oil. Toss in the escarole, parsley, and basil, season with the salt, pepper, and crushed red pepper, and cook for 2 minutes.

Remove the skins and add the whole roasted garlic cloves and the beans and simmer for 10 minutes, stirring occasionally.

For the risotto:

3 Tbsp. olive oil

2 shallots, diced

1½ cups arborio rice

6 cups vegetable stock (Pacific Natural is a gluten-
    free, low-sodium option)

¾ cup sun-dried tomatoes, cut into julienne strips

½ cup pine nuts, toasted

¼ cup vegan cream cheese

Heat the olive oil on medium-high heat in a frying or braising pan.

Add the shallots and cook for 2 to 3 minutes.

Stir in the rice, coating well.

Pour in half of the vegetable stock. Reduce the heat to
a simmer.

As the liquid reduces, add more stock about every 15
minutes. Cook until all the liquid is absorbed, about 45
minutes.

Fold in the sun-dried tomatoes, pine nuts, and cream
cheese.

Remove from the heat, cover, and set aside.

To assemble:

Place 1 cup of risotto on each plate. Top with salad greens.

Makes 6 servings.

FRENCH LENTIL AND GOLD POTATO STEW WITH FRESH HERB SALAD

For the lentils:
2 Tbsp. olive oil
⅔ cup chopped onion
½ cup diced carrot
½ cup diced celery
2 Tbsp. chopped garlic
1½ cups green lentils
4 cups vegetable stock (Pacific Natural is a gluten-
    free, low-sodium option)
1 cup diced canned tomatoes
2 bay leaves
3 sprigs fresh thyme
1 tsp. ground black pepper
Salt, to taste

Heat the oil in a pot and add the onion, carrot, and celery. Cook for 10 minutes, or until the vegetables have softened.

Add the garlic and cook for an additional minute.

Add the remaining ingredients, except for the salt. Bring to a simmer and cook, covered, for 25 to 30 minutes, or until the lentils have softened.

Season to taste with salt and set aside.

For the potatoes:
2 lb. baby gold potatoes, halved
2 tsp. salt

Place the potatoes and salt in a pot, cover with cold water, and bring to a boil. Simmer for 10 to 15 minutes, or until just tender.

Drain immediately and let cool.

For the salad:
4 cups mixed baby greens
½ cup fresh basil leaves, cut into halves or quarters
¼ cup whole flat parsley leaves, picked from the stem
¼ cup whole fresh tarragon leaves
3 Tbsp. extra-virgin olive oil
1½ Tbsp. high-quality aged balsamic or sherry wine
      vinegar
Cracked black pepper and sea salt to taste

Toss all the ingredients well to combine and season lightly with the salt and pepper.

To assemble:

Heat the potatoes together with the lentils.

Ladle about 1½ cups of the stew into serving bowls and garnish each bowl with a generous handful of the dressed salad.

Makes about 6 servings.

RED RICE AND CORN-STUFFED PEPPERS
WITH TEMPEH BACON

For the tempeh bacon:

1 (8-oz.) package tempeh, sliced lengthwise into
    thin strips

¼ cup tamari

1½ cups roasted vegetable broth (may substitute
    mushroom broth)

2 Tbsp. apple cider vinegar

1½ Tbsp. agave nectar

2 tsp. smoked paprika

½ tsp. ground coriander

½ tsp. ground cumin

½ tsp. chipotle powder

Vegetable oil

Cracked black pepper

Lay the tempeh slices in a single layer in a large, flat dish.

Combine the remaining ingredients except the oil and pepper in a saucepan, bring to a simmer, and cook for 10 minutes, or until the liquid is reduced by ¼.

Pour the hot liquid over the strips and allow the tempeh to cool in the liquid. Let marinate for 4 hours, or overnight.

Remove the tempeh from the marinade and place on a baking sheet, one layer thick.

Brush very lightly with vegetable oil, then crack fresh pepper liberally onto the exposed surface of the strips and cook in a 375°F oven for 10 to 12 minutes, or until dark brown, turning once.

Allow to cool and then dice.

For the rice and corn:
1½ cups red rice, rinsed well
½ cup small diced onion
⅓ cup diced celery
⅓ cup diced carrot
¼ cup olive oil
1 Tbsp. chopped garlic
2¼ cups vegetable broth or water
1 cup frozen corn
1 bay leaf
2 tsp. fresh marjoram
1 tsp. fresh rosemary
1 tsp. salt
1 tsp. smoked paprika (regular paprika may be substituted)
½ tsp. black pepper

In a large skillet, toast the rice over medium heat, stirring constantly for 3 to 5 minutes or until you hear popping sounds and smell the grains toasting. Remove from the heat.

In a stockpot, sauté the vegetables in the olive oil for 7 to 10 minutes, or until softened. Add the garlic and cook for an additional 3 minutes.

Add the rice and stir well.

Add the remaining ingredients, except the tempeh bacon, bring to a simmer, and cook, covered, for 15 to 20 minutes, or until the liquid is absorbed and the rice is slightly soft.*

Fold in the tempeh bacon.

Optional: Stir in 1 Tbsp. vegan butter (try Earth Balance brand)

For the peppers:
6 whole bell peppers, any color
1–2 Tbsp. extra-virgin olive oil for drizzling
Salt and freshly ground black pepper to taste

Cut the top off each pepper by carefully slicing downward just inside the lip of the pepper and at a slightly inward angle to remove the top cap.

Remove the seeds by running a knife carefully around the inside and shaking the seeds out.

Drizzle a small amount of olive oil inside and season lightly with salt and pepper.

Stuff each pepper with the cooked rice, replace the top cap, and drizzle or brush the entire outside with olive oil.

Lightly season the outside of each pepper with salt and pepper and bake at 375°F for 30 to 40 minutes, or until the pepper becomes soft and pliable.

Remove from the oven and serve immediately.

Makes 6 stuffed peppers.

CUBAN BLACK BEANS AND BROWN RICE WITH ROASTED SQUASH AND GLUTEN-FREE CRACKERS

For the rice:

2 cups brown rice
4 cups filtered water
1 bay leaf
1 tsp. sea salt

Toast the dry uncooked rice in a large, flat-bottomed sauté pan for 6 to 7 minutes, or until the rice begins to pop and emits a toasty aroma.

Place the toasted rice with the other ingredients in a pot, bring to a simmer, and cook, covered, for 45 minutes, or until the liquid is absorbed and the rice has softened.

Stir to fluff and reserve.

For the beans:

2 Tbsp. olive oil
½ cup diced onion
½ cup diced carrot
1 green or yellow bell pepper, seeded and diced
1 Tbsp. chopped garlic
1½ tsp. chili powder
½ tsp. cumin
1 (14.5-oz.) can diced tomatoes
3½ cups cooked, drained black beans
¼ cup chopped fresh cilantro
Salt and black pepper, to taste

Heat the oil in a pot.

Add the onion, carrot, and pepper and cook for 10 to 12 minutes, or until softened.

Add the garlic and cook for 1 minute.

Add the dry spices and cook for another minute.

Add the tomatoes and simmer for 3 minutes.

Add the remaining ingredients and heat through.

To assemble:
2 zucchini
2 yellow squash
2 tsp. olive oil
Salt and pepper to taste

Slice the zucchini and squash into ½-inch-thick rounds on a slight angle to form elongated ovals.

Brush both sides with the oil and sprinkle with salt and pepper.

Place on a cookie sheet in a single layer and roast for 12 minutes, or until softened, in a 375°F oven.

Serve the beans over the rice with some of the vegetables and Mary's Gone Crackers or Edward & Sons gluten-free crackers.

Makes 5 to 6 servings.

GLUTEN-FREE TABOULEH OVER BABY GREENS WITH CRUNCHY ALMONDS

For the tabouleh:
1½ cups quinoa
3 cups water
1 tsp. sea salt

Place the ingredients in a saucepan, bring to a simmer, and cook, covered, for 20 minutes, or until the liquid has been absorbed and the grain has softened.

Stir once, spread out onto a cookie sheet, and let cool completely.

For the almonds:
½ cup sliced almonds
Sprinkle of sea salt

Place the almond slices on a cookie sheet in a thin layer.

Sprinkle lightly with the sea salt.

Place in a 375°F oven and cook for 12 minutes, or until lightly browned, stirring once. Set aside.

For the salad:
Cooked quinoa
2 cups grape tomatoes, halved
⅔ cup chopped flat-leaf parsley
5 green onions, sliced thinly
1 English cucumber, peeled and diced
Juice of 2 lemons (about ⅔ cup)

⅓ cup extra-virgin olive oil

1 tsp. or more sea salt, to taste

1½ tsp. black pepper

3 cups fairly loosely packed baby greens

Combine all the ingredients except the baby greens in a large bowl and mix well.

Arrange the baby greens on 6 large plates.

Scoop about 1½ cups of the tabouleh over the greens, sprinkle with the toasted almonds, and serve with gluten-free crackers, such as Mary's Gone Crackers Black Pepper Crackers.

Makes 6 salads.

Bavarian Tempeh with Shaved Fennel Salad and Quinoa Timbale

For the tempeh:

3 (8-oz.) packages tempeh

3 cups water

1 cup chopped prunes

3-inch piece ginger, cut into 6 pieces

½ cup apple cider vinegar

1 orange, cut into 4 segments

Slice the tempeh on an angle into ½ inch slices.

Lay in a single layer in a flat-bottomed pan.

Add all the remaining ingredients and cook over medium-high heat.

Bring to a simmer, adjusting the heat to maintain a simmer for 30 minutes.

Carefully transfer the tempeh to a dish and set aside.

Strain the cooking liquid, return the juice to low heat, and let reduce for an additional 15 minutes.

For the fennel slaw layer:

1½ lb. fresh fennel, shaved very thinly

1 cup julienne carrots

2 Tbsp. fresh lemon juice

1 Tbsp. extra-virgin olive oil

1 Tbsp. chopped fresh dill

½ tsp. finely grated fresh lemon zest

⅛ tsp. salt

Mix all the ingredients together in a large bowl. Set aside.

For the quinoa layer:

1 cup quinoa

2 cups vegetable stock (Pacific Natural is a gluten-free, low-sodium option)

1 Tbsp. extra-virgin olive oil

1 Tbsp. diced red onion

Cook the quinoa in the stock over medium heat until translucent.

Let cool. Add the olive oil and the red onion. Set aside.

To assemble:

1 Tbsp. arrowroot

1 Tbsp. cold water

1 cup canned mandarin orange segments, drained

Mix the arrowroot and cold water to form a slurry. Stir into the reducing tempeh stock to thicken the liquid. Add the mandarin orange segments.

Place a few drops of olive oil in a ½ cup measuring cup and coat the inside. Pack some of the quinoa into the cup. Turn the cup over onto a plate and tap out the quinoa.

Return the tempeh to the thickened liquid for a few minutes to warm.

Place the tempeh on plates with the quinoa and garnish with the fennel slaw.

Spoon some sauce and orange segments over the tempeh and serve.

Makes 6 servings.

CREAMY SQUASH SOUP WITH TOASTED ALMOND SLICES

For the almonds:

⅓ cup raw sliced almonds

Place the almond slices in a 350°F oven and toast for 10 to 12 minutes, stirring once, until golden brown.

Remove from the oven and reserve.

For the soup:
1 Tbsp. vegan butter (try Earth Balance brand)
½ medium onion, diced
1 1-inch peeled piece fresh ginger, minced
1 clove garlic, minced
½ medium butternut squash, peeled, seeded, and
    cubed
2 sprigs fresh thyme
1 bay leaf
½ Tbsp. chopped fresh sage
About ¾ quart vegetable broth (1 container Pacific
    Natural Vegetable Broth)
1 Tbsp. arrowroot
1 Tbsp. cold water
Salt and pepper, to taste

Heat the vegan butter in a medium saucepan and sauté the onion until soft. Add the ginger and garlic and mix.

Add the butternut squash, thyme sprigs, bay leaf, sage, and just enough broth to cover the squash. Cover and bring to a boil. Turn the heat down and simmer for about 30 minutes, or until the squash is soft.

Mix the arrowroot with the cold water in a separate bowl to make a slurry and drizzle into the soup while stirring constantly.

Simmer for an additional 5 minutes.

Put the mixture into a blender or use an immersion blender to blend until smooth. Season with salt and pepper. Garnish each soup with a small amount of the toasted almonds.

Makes 6 to 7 servings.

Tamari-Baked Tofu over Mixed Greens with Sweet Onions and Balsamic Dressing

For the tofu:
2 lb. extra-firm tofu, drained well
¼ cup wheat-free tamari
2 Tbsp. olive oil
1 tsp. toasted sesame oil
1 tsp. minced ginger

Slice the tofu into 3 or 4 slices lengthwise, place in a pan with holes or a strainer and press out the water gently with a clean towel. Press several times and allow the tofu to drain for 2 to 3 hours.

Slice the blocks into long, thin rectangles of about 3 inches in length and ½ inch in cross section.

Mix all the other ingredients well in a bowl.

Place the tofu one layer think on a cookie sheet and pour the marinade on top.

Cook in a preheated 375°F oven for 20 to 25 minutes, turning once, or until the tofu has browned well and the liquid begins to caramelize.

Remove from the oven and cool in the liquid.

For the salad:
6 fairly loosely packed cups baby greens (any
    varietal will work: baby spinach, baby romaine,
    radicchio, frisée, red leaf, etc.)
1 cup sliced teardrop tomatoes

1 cup thinly sliced sweet onion

¼ cup whole basil leaves, cut into large pieces

¼ cup whole fresh tarragon leaves

⅓ cup extra-virgin olive oil

3 Tbsp. aged balsamic vinegar

½ tsp. salt

Cracked black pepper, to taste

Combine the greens, tomatoes, onion, basil, and tarragon, and toss well.

Add the oil, vinegar, salt, and pepper, and toss to just moisten the leaves.

Place on 6 or 7 dinner plates, distribute the tofu pieces evenly among the plates, and serve.

Optional: Serve with gluten-free crackers.

Makes 6 or 7 large salads.

TOMATO AND ONION QUESADILLAS WITH
FRESH GUACAMOLE AND VEGAN SOUR CREAM

For the guacamole:

4 large avocados, peeled, pits removed

1 red bell pepper, seeded and diced

½ cup diced red onion

3 Tbsp. chopped cilantro

1 tsp. minced garlic

1 jalapeño pepper, seeded and minced

1 tsp. salt or to taste

Mash the avocados to form a paste, then add the remaining ingredients and adjust the seasoning with the salt.

For the quesadillas:
6 to 8 large beefsteak tomatoes
3 Tbsp. olive oil
1 Tbsp. chili powder
1½ Tbsp. salt
2 tsp. ground coriander
1 tsp. ground cumin
1 tsp. chipotle powder
3 large yellow onions, halved and sliced into large, rough slices
2 Tbsp. vegetable oil
1 Tbsp. garlic
1 tsp. salt
1 Tbsp. cracked black pepper
16 gluten-free tortillas (try Don Pancho brand) 6-inch size
2 (10-oz.) packages vegan nacho- or cheddar-flavored cheese, shredded (try Follow Your Heart brand)
Oil for brushing the quesadillas
1 (8-oz.) container vegan sour cream (try Follow Your Heart brand)

Slice the tomatoes into large, ¼-inch slabs. Place one-layer thick on cookie sheets and brush with the olive oil.

Combine the dry spices and sprinkle over the tomato slices. Bake at 425°F for 10 to 15 minutes, or until softened.

Cook the onions in the vegetable oil over medium heat until caramelized, about 15 minutes. Be sure to cook the onions until golden brown, then add the garlic, salt, and pepper and cook for an additional minute.

Place eight tortillas on a work surface and distribute the tomatoes, cooked onions, and grated "cheese" evenly among them.

Cover with the remaining tortillas and brush the tops of the quesadillas lightly with oil. Cook, oiled-side down, in a large sauté pan or griddle over medium-high heat for 3 minutes.

Brush the exposed side of each quesadilla lightly with oil, then flip and cook the second side for 3 minutes, or until heated through.

Slice each into four segments and serve with the fresh guacamole and vegan sour cream.

Makes 8 quesadillas

VEGAN PAD THAI WITH SHIITAKE MUSHROOMS

1 lb. wide rice noodles, dry
6 Tbsp. gluten-free reduced-sodium tamari or
    soy sauce
2 Tbsp. agave nectar
Juice of 1 lime
¾ tsp. red-pepper flakes
¼ cup vegetable oil
2 cups sliced shiitake mushrooms
2 Tbsp. chopped garlic
2 tsp. minced fresh ginger

1 lb. extra-firm tofu, drained and cut into ½-inch
  cubes
2 cups bean sprouts
1 cup chopped peanuts
⅔ cup cilantro leaves
½ cup sliced green onions
2 Tbsp. toasted sesame oil

Soak the noodles in cold water for 30 minutes, or until softened. Drain and set aside.

Cook the softened noodles in rapidly boiling water according to the package directions (about 1 to 4 minutes),
drain, and set aside.

Combine the agave, lime juice, and pepper flakes, and
reserve.

Heat the oil in a wok or large sauté pan and stir-fry the
mushrooms for 3 to 5 minutes, or until softened.

Add the garlic, ginger, and tofu and cook until heated
through, about 2 minutes.

Add all the remaining ingredients and quickly stir-fry
to heat the noodles completely through, about 3 minutes,
and serve.

Makes 8 to 10 servings.

DINNERS

SPAGHETTI WITH PESTO CREAM

For the pesto:
2 cups fresh basil leaves
½ cup pine nuts
3 garlic cloves
3 Tbsp. nutritional yeast
1 Tbsp. white miso paste
⅓ cup extra-virgin olive oil
1½ tsp. salt
Cracked black pepper, to taste

Place the basil, pine nuts, garlic, yeast, and miso, in a food processor and pulse several times to create a coarse mixture.

Add the olive oil a little bit at a time, over four or five additional pulses, and then season with the salt and cracked pepper and reserve.

For the pasta:
1½ tsp. rice flour
⅓ cup cold organic coconut milk
⅓ cup vegetable broth
1½ lbs. gluten-free rice pasta (try Mrs. Leeper's brand)
1½ pints cherry tomatoes, halved
3 cups baby spinach

Mix the rice flour well into the cold coconut milk and vegetable broth, bring to a simmer, and cook for about 5 minutes, or until thickened.

Cook the pasta according to the package directions, drain, and add to the thickened, simmering sauce.

Fold in the tomatoes and baby spinach and heat through.

Fold in the pesto and carefully heat through, being careful not to boil the sauce.

Makes 8 to 10 servings.

Black Bean, Avocado, and Corn Salad with Blackened Tofu

For the salad:
1 (15-oz.) can black beans, drained and rinsed
1 avocado, peeled, pit removed, diced
3 tomatoes, seeded and diced into ½-inch pieces
1 cup frozen corn kernels, defrosted
1 Tbsp. chopped cilantro
½ tsp. cumin
½ tsp. salt
2 romaine hearts

Mix together all the ingredients except for the romaine and refrigerate.

Rinse the romaine hearts, drain, and dice into 1-inch pieces. Set both the salad and the romaine pieces aside.

For the dressing:
¼ cup fresh lime juice (about 2 limes)
½ cup vegetable oil
1 Tbsp. seeded and minced jalapeño
3 Tbsp. vegan cream cheese

1 Tbsp. agave nectar
½ tsp. salt

Place the lime juice in a small mixing bowl. Using a wire whisk, slowly whip in the oil in a slow stream.

Add the diced jalapeños and whip in the vegan cream cheese, agave, and salt. Mix well, creating a smooth dressing.

For the tofu:
1 (14-oz.) package extra-firm tofu, cut into 6½-inch-thick pieces, pressed between paper towels, and patted dry
2 Tbsp. olive oil
3 Tbsp. blackened seasoning (try Chef Paul Prudhomme's Magic Seasoning blend)

Cut the tofu sections in half from corner to corner, forming long triangles.

Pour the olive oil into a shallow baking dish.

Coat the tofu in the olive oil and sprinkle with half of the blackened seasoning. Transfer to a plate, seasoned side down. Coat with the remaining seasoning.

Place a heavy iron skillet or thick-bottomed sauté pan over high heat for about 5 minutes.

Place the tofu pieces in the pan and cook for 3 to 4 minutes on each side.

To assemble:
Pour half the dressing into the black bean and avocado salad and toss.

Place the romaine on a plate and top with 1 cup of the black bean and avocado salad. Top with three tofu rectangles.

Drizzle the remaining dressing on top of the tofu and lettuce.

Makes 4 servings.

ROASTED SUMMER CORN AND BASIL GRITS WITH BLACK BEAN CHIPOTLE BURGER AND SPROUTS

For the corn:
4 ears yellow sweet corn

Remove the silky hairs from the tops of the corn ears, but leave husks intact.

Place the ears on a baking sheet and roast in a 425°F oven for 20 minutes, or until the husks begin to brown and the kernels have softened (to test, peel back one ear to expose some kernels and poke with a fork; if they pierce easily and hot liquid oozes out, they are done).

Allow for cooling, then remove the husks and hairs completely.

Over a large, clean towel (to catch stray kernels), remove the kernels from the cob by cutting down the cob with a sharp knife.

For the grits:
5 cups water
2 tsp. salt
1 cup hominy (white corn) grits (not instant)

6 Gardenburger black bean chipotle burgers
    (defrosted)
2 Tbsp. vegan butter (try Earth Balance brand)
    ¼ cup chopped fresh basil
Salt and black pepper, to taste
1 cup sprouts (dandelion, alfalfa, or any other
    varietal will work)

Place the water and salt in a pot, bring to a simmer, and carefully add the grits.

Bring back to a simmer and cook for 20 to 25 minutes, stirring often, or until the grits have softened. (Note: Use package directions for cooking the grits if you wish—also, once the grits become thick, they may start bubbling out of the pot if the heat is too high; reduce the heat and stir more often if this begins to happen.)

While the grits are cooking, place the burger patties in a 350°F oven on a baking sheet until heated through, about 10 minutes.

Cut the burger patties into three or four slices and keep warm.

Add the roasted corn kernels to the grits and heat through.

Remove from the heat and quickly swirl in the vegan butter and the basil. Season to taste with salt and pepper.

Ladle the cooked grits into six serving bowls, then top with the heated burger patties and finally with a generous garnish of the fresh sprouts.

Makes 6 entrée servings.

OLD BAY TOFU CAKES WITH CREAMY HORSERADISH AND CREOLE MUSTARD SAUCE OVER SHAVED FENNEL SLAW

For the fennel slaw:
1½ lbs. fresh fennel, shaved very thinly
1 cup julienne carrots
1 Tbsp. chopped fresh dill
2 Tbsp. fresh lemon juice
1 Tbsp. extra-virgin olive oil
½ tsp. finely grated fresh lemon zest
⅛ tsp. salt

Mix all the ingredients together in a large bowl. Set aside.

For the sauce:
¾ cup vegan mayonnaise (try Vegenaise)
¾ cup vegan sour cream (try Follow Your Heart brand)
2½ Tbsp. bottled horseradish
2 Tbsp. coarsely ground Creole mustard
Juice of 1 lemon (about 1½ Tbsp.)
2 tsp. sea salt
Freshly cracked black pepper to taste

Combine all the ingredients except the pepper in a bowl and mix well.

Adjust the seasoning with black pepper.

Refrigerate until ready to serve.

For the cakes:
½ cup finely diced onion
½ cup finely diced carrot
2 Tbsp vegetable oil
2 tsp. minced garlic
2 lb. firm tofu
¼ cup nutritional yeast
2½ Tbsp. cornstarch
1 Tbsp. salt
½ tsp. ground white pepper
Juice of 1 lime

Sauté the onion and carrot in the oil until soft, about 3 to 5 minutes.

Add the garlic and sauté for 1 minute longer. Let cool completely.

Add the remaining ingredients, mix well, and let cool in the refrigerator for 30 minutes.

To assemble:
2 cups brown-rice flour
3 Tbsp. Old Bay seasoning
1 tsp. salt
1½ cups unsweetened soy milk
Canola oil

Mix the rice flour, Old Bay, and salt together.

Form small, approximately 2-ounce, cakes from the tofu mixture by hand.

Immerse each cake in the soy milk.

Dredge the cakes in the seasoned flour, coating each well. Refrigerate the cakes for 30 minutes to set firm.

Sauté at medium-high heat in vegetable oil (make certain that oil is about halfway up the side of each cake) until browned on both sides and heated completely through.

Serve the cakes over a small amount of the slaw and top with the sauce.

Optional: Place ⅔ cup baby greens on the plate, then the slaw on top.

Makes 12 to 14 cakes.

BLACK-BEAN CAKES WITH LIME-PEPPERED "MAYO"

For the black-bean cakes:

30 oz. cooked black beans, rinsed and drained

¼ cup bread crumbs made from wheat-free bread

2 Tbsp. vegan butter, softened (try Earth Balance brand)

2 Tbsp. chopped cilantro

2 Tbsp. chopped shallots

2 tsp. minced garlic

2 tsp. Creole seasoning

Salt and pepper to taste

¼ cup canola oil

Preheat the oven to 300°F.

Place the beans on paper towels to soak up the excess moisture. Bake the beans on a cookie sheet for 20 minutes. Let cool.

In a food processor, combine the beans, bread crumbs, vegan butter, cilantro, shallots, garlic, Creole seasoning, salt, and pepper. Refrigerate for 1 to 2 hours.

Form the bean mixture into patties. Heat the oil in a skillet over medium heat. Fry the cakes for 4 minutes, until browned and crispy, then flip and cook on the other side. Drain on paper towels.

For the lime-peppered "mayo":
1 cup vegan mayonnaise (try Vegenaise)
1½ tsp. fresh lime juice
1 jalapeño pepper, minced
Salt and pepper, to taste

Mix the vegan mayonnaise, the lime juice, and the jalapeño in a bowl. Season with the salt and pepper and refrigerate until ready to serve. Serve with the black bean cakes.

Makes 6 to 7 servings

ROASTED JAPANESE EGGPLANT AND SQUASH WITH FRESH BASIL AND FIRE-ROASTED TOMATO SAUCE WITH QUINOA

For the sauce:
¼ cup extra-virgin olive oil
1 medium onion, diced
3 cloves garlic, chopped
2 (28-oz.) cans Muir Glen fire roasted diced
   tomatoes

1 (14.5-oz.) can Muir Glen fire roasted crushed
   tomatoes
⅔ cup vegetable stock (Pacific Natural is a gluten-
   free, low-sodium option)
⅓ cup chopped fresh basil
1 Tbsp. agave nectar
1 Tbsp. coarse-ground black pepper
2 tsp. salt

Heat the oil in a saucepan.

Sauté the onion in the oil for 5 to 7 minutes, or until softened.

Add the garlic and cook for an additional minute.

Add the tomatoes and stock and bring to a simmer, cooking for 25 minutes.

Add the basil, agave, pepper, and salt, and set aside.

For the quinoa:
4 cups water
2 cups quinoa
1 tsp. sea salt

Place all the ingredients in a stockpot and simmer for 15 to 20 minutes, or until the grain has softened.

Drain any excess liquid.

For the vegetables:
4 or 5 Japanese eggplants
2 yellow squash

2 zucchini
⅓ cup olive oil
Salt and black pepper, to taste
⅓ cup micro greens or sprouts (optional garnish)

Slice all the vegetables on a slight diagonal into ¼-inch-thick slices.

Brush each side with olive oil, sprinkle with salt and pepper, and roast on a cookie sheet in a preheated 375°F oven for 12 minutes, or until the vegetables just begin to soften.

To serve:

Place about 1½ cups of cooked, hot quinoa on each plate. Ladle ⅔ cup of the sauce on top and arrange the heated spears of cooked vegetables over the entire plate.

Garnish with the micro greens or sprouts, if using.

Makes approximately 6 servings.

WILD MUSHROOM, PERUVIAN POTATO, AND BABY GREENS WITH TOFU

For the potatoes:
2 lb. purple Peruvian potatoes, diced
2 tsp. sea salt

Place the potatoes and salt in a pot, cover with water, and simmer for 15 to 20 minutes, or until just softened.

Drain well and reserve.

For the mushrooms, tofu, and greens:

¼ cup olive oil

3 cups sliced wild mushrooms (any varietals will
    work: shiitake, cremini, blue foot, chanterelle,
    oyster, hen of the woods, etc.)

4 cups baby greens (spinach, stemmed and rinsed
    dandelion, or any other hearty baby green will
    work), washed well

2 cloves garlic, chopped

1 lb. extra-firm tofu, drained well and cut into ½-
    inch dice

1 tsp. fresh thyme, chopped

1 Tbsp. cracked black pepper

1½ tsp. sea salt

1½ Tbsp. vegan butter (try Earth Balance brand)

Heat the oil in a large sauté pan.

Add the mushrooms and sauté on high heat for 5 minutes, or until softened.

Add the greens and garlic and sauté for 3 minutes, or until the greens have just begun to wilt.

Add the remaining ingredients, including the potatoes, except for the vegan butter, and heat through.

Remove from the heat, stir in the vegan butter, and serve immediately.

Makes about 4 servings.

Chimichurri Tofu and Mushroom Skewers
over Sweet Chili Rice

For the skewers:

1 package extra-firm tofu
1½ cups flat parsley, washed
¼ cup red-wine vinegar
6 cloves garlic
1 Tbsp. chopped red onion
1½ tsp. lemon juice
1 tsp. salt
¾ tsp. red-pepper flakes
½ cup extra-virgin olive oil
8–12 wooden skewers
1 whole red bell pepper, seeded and cut into 1-inch
    squares
1 yellow bell pepper, seeded and cut into 1-inch
    squares
1 pint whole cherry tomatoes
1 lb. whole cremini mushrooms, stems removed

Remove the tofu from the package and press well into a clean cloth to remove excess liquid.

Slice the tofu into 1-inch cubes and set aside.

Place the parsley, vinegar, garlic, onion, lemon juice, salt, and red-pepper flakes in a food processor and blend to form a paste.

Slowly add the oil to form a pesto-like paste.

Skewer the tofu cubes, peppers, tomatoes, and mushrooms alternately to form kebabs.

Place the skewers in a large baking dish, forming one flat layer.

Slather both sides of the skewers well with the marinade, cover, and let sit for 4 hours or overnight.

Using a charcoal grill or a grill pan, grill the skewers for 3 to 5 minutes on each side, or until well marked and heated through.

For the rice:
2 Tbsp. vegetable oil
½ cup chopped onion
2 tsp. chopped garlic
1 red bell pepper, seeded and diced
1 yellow bell pepper, seeded and diced
1 poblano pepper, seeded and diced
3 cups water
1½ cups brown rice
1 bay leaf
2 tsp. salt
1 Tbsp. vegan butter (try Earth Balance brand)

Heat the oil in a pot and add the onion, cooking for 5 to 7 minutes, or until softened.

Add the garlic and cook for an additional minute.

Add the diced peppers, water, rice, bay leaf, and salt, and bring to a simmer.

Cook, covered, for 25 to 35 minutes, or until all the liquid is absorbed and the rice is softened.

Fold in the vegan butter and serve with the skewers on top.

Makes 8 to 12 servings.

GRILLED CUBAN-STYLE SUNSHINE BURGERS

For the dry rub:
1 Tbsp. sea salt
1 tsp. ground black pepper
1 tsp. garlic powder
1 tsp. onion powder
1 tsp. ground cumin
1 tsp. dry oregano
1 tsp. dry thyme
1 tsp. smoked paprika
¼ tsp. cayenne pepper
2 Sunshine (or other gluten-free) veggie burgers
Olive oil

Combine all the ingredients except the veggie burgers in a mortar and pestle or spice grinder.

Rub the burgers with olive oil and sprinkle with the dry rub. Brown on each side in a cast-iron skillet, grill, or sauté pan.

For the sofrito:
2 Tbsp. olive oil
1 red bell pepper, diced small
1 red onion, diced small
3 garlic cloves, minced

1 (8-oz.) can diced tomatoes
3 Tbsp. chopped parsley
1 tsp. smoked paprika
Salt and pepper to taste

Heat the olive oil in a sauté pan and sauté the peppers, onion, and garlic for 4 to 5 minutes. Add the tomatoes, parsley, and paprika. Season with salt and pepper and continue to cook for 10 minutes.

Serve the burgers with sliced avocado and top with the sofrito.

Makes 2 servings.

ARTICHOKE AND SHIITAKE MUSHROOM PAELLA

For the sofrito:
2 Tbsp. olive oil
1 red bell pepper, diced small
1 red onion, diced small
3 garlic cloves, minced
1 (8-oz.) can diced tomatoes
3 Tbsp. chopped parsley
1 tsp. smoked paprika
Salt and pepper, to taste

Heat the olive oil in a sauté pan and sauté the peppers, onion, and garlic for 4 to 5 minutes. Add the tomatoes, parsley, and paprika. Season with salt and pepper and continue to cook for 10 minutes.

For the rice:
1 cup rice
3 cups vegetable stock (Pacific Natural is a gluten-
    free, low-sodium option)
Pinch of saffron
1½ tsp. salt
½ tsp. pepper
1 cup frozen peas

Add the rice to the pan with the sofrito and cook for
1 minute. Add the stock and saffron and season with the
salt and pepper. Cook on medium-high heat for 8 minutes,
then reduce the heat and simmer, uncovered, for 15 to 20
minutes, or until the liquid has evaporated and the rice is
tender

During the last 5 minutes of cooking, pour the peas over
the rice and let steam. When the rice is done cooking, stir
everything together.

For the toppings:
2 Tbsp. olive oil
4 oz. shiitake mushrooms, stems removed, halved or
    quartered depending on size
1 (8-oz.) can artichoke hearts, drained and cut in half
Salt and pepper, to taste
2 Tbsp. fresh lemon juice

Heat the oil in a medium sauté pan and sauté the mushrooms
and artichoke hearts over medium heat, stirring often, for
about 10 minutes or until browned on each side. Season with

salt and pepper, then turn off the heat and stir in the lemon juice.

Serve on top of the rice.

Makes 3 to 4 servings.

Mushrooms and Garlic Greens over Broiled Polenta, Tofu, and Tomatoes

For the mushrooms and greens:
¼ cup olive oil
2½ cups sliced mushrooms (any varietal will work: cremini, button, shiitake, trumpet, blue foot, etc.)
½ lb. braising greens (turnip, collard, mustard, Swiss chard, spinach, etc.), stems removed, washed thoroughly, and roughly chopped into large squares
1½ Tbsp. chopped garlic
2 tsp. salt
1 tsp. black pepper

Heat the oil in a large, flat-bottomed skillet and sauté the mushrooms for 7 to 8 minutes, or until softened.

Add the greens and garlic and quickly wilt over high heat for about 3 minutes, or until the greens begin to weep their liquid and soften.

Season with the salt and pepper and set aside.

For the polenta, tofu, and tomatoes:
1 (1½-lb.) package San Gennaro (or other equivalent brand) prepared polenta

1 lb. extra-firm tofu
2 large ripe tomatoes
4 Tbsp. extra-virgin olive oil
1½ Tbsp. chopped rosemary
Salt and cracked black pepper to taste

Slice the polenta into eight even slices, about ½ inch thick.

Drain the tofu, slice lengthwise into 4 thin blocks, and press lightly between two clean cloths to drain excess water.

Cut the tomatoes into eight slices roughly equal to the polenta (this may require more than two tomatoes, depending on their size).

Brush the polenta, tofu, and tomato slices with the oil, sprinkle with the rosemary, and season lightly with salt and freshly cracked pepper on both sides.

Place the tofu and polenta slices on a baking sheet. Place the tomatoes on another baking sheet (using two baking sheets is a good idea because the tomatoes will probably be done before the tofu and polenta). Broil for about 7 to 8 minutes, turning once, or until browned and heated through.

Remove from the oven. Place two polenta slices on a plate, followed by one tofu slice and two tomato slices. Top with a generous portion of the mushrooms and greens to finish the plate.

Makes 4 large entrées.

CORN FRITTERS WITH FRESH GUACAMOLE

For the guacamole:
2 medium ripe avocados, peeled, pits removed,
      and diced
2 garlic cloves, minced
Juice of 1 lemon
1 Tbsp. minced jalapeño
Salt to taste
¼ cup diced tomato

In a large bowl, combine the avocados, garlic, lemon juice, and jalapeño. Season with salt. Gently stir in the diced tomato, cover, and refrigerate until serving.

For the fritters:
3 ears of corn, shucked and kernels removed
¼ cup soy milk
2 Tbsp. cornstarch
½ cup plus 1 Tbsp. vegetable oil
3 large shiitake mushrooms (2 oz.), stems discarded
      and caps cut into ½-inch dice
¼ cup diced sweet onion
½ cup corn flour
¼ cup cornmeal
1 tsp. baking powder
1½ tsp. salt
½ tsp. black pepper

Place half the corn kernels into a blender. Scrape the pulp from the cobs into the blender. Add the soy milk and cornstarch. Purée until smooth.

In a large nonstick skillet, heat the 1 Tbsp. of oil. Add the shiitakes and onion and cook over high heat, stirring occasionally, until lightly browned, about 5 minutes. Add the remaining corn and cook, stirring, for 1 minute. Transfer to a plate and place in the freezer for about 5 minutes, until no longer hot.

In a bowl, whisk together the flour, cornmeal, baking powder, salt, and pepper. Stir in the purée, and then fold in the cooled corn mixture.

Wipe out the skillet. Add ¼ cup of oil and heat over medium-high heat. When hot, add four level, ¼-cup mounds of batter to the skillet and spread each to a ½-inch thickness. Fry, turning once, until golden and crusty, about 4 minutes. Repeat with remaining oil and batter. Drain on paper towels and serve warm, topped with guacamole.

Makes 2 to 3 servings.

Gnocchi Tossed with a Mushroom Cream Sauce

For the gnocchi:
1 lb. white potatoes, peeled and quartered
2 oz. silken tofu, mashed or puréed
2 Tbsp. chickpea flour
2 Tbsp. potato starch
Sea salt to taste

Place the potatoes in a large pot filled with salted water. Bring to a boil over high heat and let cook for about 20 minutes, or until tender.

Drain the potatoes and then put into a large bowl. Mash until smooth.

Sprinkle the tofu, flour, and starch into the bowl with one hand while kneading it into the potatoes with the other. Continue until it just forms a smooth dough.

Divide the dough into three pieces. Form the dough into a 1- to 2-inch-thick roll. Cut the roll into inch-long sections and press each with the tines of a fork. Repeat with the remaining dough.

Drop the gnocchi, one at a time, into heavily salted boiling water. Cook for 2 to 3 minutes, or until they rise to the surface.

Remove the gnocchi from the water, drain well, and set aside.

For the sauce:
2 Tbsp. vegan butter (try Earth Balance brand)
8–12 oz. shiitake mushrooms, sliced
1 clove garlic, minced
1¼ cups unsweetened soy milk
1 Tbsp. cornstarch
1 Tbsp. chopped fresh parsley
Juice of ½ lemon
Salt and pepper to taste

Melt 1 Tbsp. of the vegan butter in a sauté pan. Add the mushrooms and garlic and sauté until soft, about 4 to 5 minutes. Remove from the pan and set aside.

Add the remaining tablespoon of vegan butter to the pan and, when melted, pour in the soy milk. Gradually whisk in the cornstarch.

Add the mushrooms, parsley, lemon juice, salt, and pepper, and cook for 1 to 2 minutes, or until thickened.

Toss with the cooked gnocchi and serve immediately.

Makes 4 servings.

BLACKENED TOFU AND AVOCADO TACOS

1 (16-oz.) package extra-firm tofu

1 Tbsp. paprika

2 tsp. black pepper

1½ tsp. salt

1 tsp. garlic powder

1 tsp. cayenne pepper

1 tsp. chipotle pepper

2 Tbsp. olive oil

8 corn tortillas

1 ripe avocado, pitted and sliced

½ tomato, diced

¼ red onion, thinly sliced

1 lime, cut into wedges

Vegan sour cream for garnish (try Follow Your Heart brand)

Salsa for garnish

Drain the tofu, pat dry with a towel or paper towel, and then cut into four equal-size pieces.

In a small bowl, combine the paprika, pepper, salt, garlic powder, cayenne, and chipotle.

Dip all sides of each piece of the tofu into the blackened seasoning.

Heat the olive oil in a pan over medium-high heat. Add the tofu and cook on each side about 5 to 7 minutes, or until a crust begins to form.

While cooking the tofu, preheat the oven to 350°F. Wrap the corn tortillas in foil and place in the oven until warm, not crispy, about 7 minutes.

Remove the tofu from the heat and slice into strips.

Top each tortilla with tofu strips, avocado slices, tomato, onion, and lime juice.

Garnish with vegan sour cream and salsa.

Makes 4 servings.

TOMATO HERB RISOTTO

2 Tbsp. olive oil

1 cup chopped onion

6 cups vegetable stock (Pacific Natural is a gluten-free, low-sodium option)

1 tsp. chopped garlic

2 cups arborio rice

Juice of 1 lemon

2 Tbsp. red-wine vinegar

1 tsp. agave nectar

¼ cup extra-virgin olive oil

½ cup cherry or grape tomatoes, quartered
¼ cup red onion, diced
2 Tbsp. mint, chopped
2 Tbsp. basil, chopped
Salt and pepper to taste

Heat the oil in a large sauté pan over medium-low heat. Add the onion and sauté until slightly soft, about 3 minutes.

Add the stock and garlic. Bring the mixture to a boil, reduce the heat to medium, and simmer for about 6 minutes.

Add the rice and simmer for 20 minutes, stirring constantly. During final 5 minutes of cooking, reduce the heat to low. Cook until the rice is tender and creamy and the liquid has evaporated or been absorbed.

To make the vinaigrette, whisk together the lemon juice, vinegar, and agave nectar in a small bowl and slowly add the oil while stirring continuously.

Add the vinaigrette, tomatoes, onion, mint, and basil to the risotto and simmer for an additional 2 minutes, stirring constantly. Season with salt and pepper.

Makes 4 to 6 servings.

FRESH HERB-BRAISED TEMPEH WITH ASPARAGUS AND WHITE BEAN AND WILD MUSHROOM MASH

For the tempeh:
1 stalk celery, washed and roughly chopped
1 medium carrot, peeled and roughly chopped
½ sweet onion, peeled and roughly chopped
5 sprigs fresh thyme

2 sprigs fresh rosemary

2 bay leaves

2 Tbsp. salt

2 Tbsp. whole black peppercorns

3 cups water

3 (8-oz.) packages tempeh

Combine all the ingredients, except the tempeh, in a large, flat-bottomed pan. Bring to a simmer and cook for 10 minutes, allowing the flavors to develop.

Slice the tempeh across the width, on an angle, into 1-inch by 2-inch slices.

Place the tempeh in the simmering liquid and cook for 20 minutes, or until softened.

Remove the tempeh from the liquid and save the liquid, with the vegetables and herbs still in the sauce.

For the bean mash:

3 Tbsp. olive oil

2 cups exotic mushrooms (any varietal will work: cremini, shiitake, chanterelle, blue foot, etc.), stems removed and sliced into thin slivers

2 cloves garlic, minced

4 (6-oz.) cans cooked white beans, rinsed and drained very well

2 Tbsp. vegan butter (try Earth Balance brand)

Salt and cracked black pepper, to taste

Heat the oil in a large sauté pan and sauté the mushrooms for 7 to 8 minutes, or until softened.

Add the garlic and cook for 2 more minutes.

Add the drained beans and heat through.

Transfer to a bowl, add the vegan butter, and mash with a potato masher or the back of a large spoon to create a rough paste.

Season with salt and pepper and keep warm.

For the asparagus:
2 large bunches asparagus
1 tsp. salt

Cut off the tough ends of the asparagus and cut the asparagus into segments about 1 inch long.

Bring a medium-size pot of water to a boil. Add the salt.

Add the asparagus and cook for 5 minutes, or until just soft but still crisp.

Immediately drain and plunge the segments into a bowl of ice water to rapidly cool and to preserve the green color.

Drain and reserve.

To assemble:
2 Tbsp. arrowroot or cornstarch
2 Tbsp. cold water
1½ Tbsp. vegan butter (try Earth Balance brand)
Salt and freshly cracked black pepper to taste
1 large red bell pepper
1 large yellow bell pepper
¼ cup finely chopped chives for garnish

Bring the cooking liquid from the tempeh to a simmer.

Combine the arrowroot and cold water to form a thick paste.

Quickly swirl the arrowroot paste into the simmering liquid and cook for 3 minutes to thicken.

Remove from the heat, swirl in the vegan butter to form a creamy sauce, and immediately strain through a fine-mesh strainer into a clean pot for the finished sauce.

Season with salt and pepper.

Cut the ends off the bell peppers, slice each in half, and remove the seeds. Carefully cut away as much of the white ribs as possible, then slice each half into very thin, long strips and place in a bowl of ice water while finishing the dish.

Briefly reheat the asparagus spears and tempeh in the sauce and place about ¾ cup of the bean mash onto 5 plates.

Place pieces of the cooked tempeh on top of the beans and place some asparagus spears around the outside of the beans.

Ladle the sauce on top.

Pull the peppers out of the ice bath (if sliced thinly enough, they should curl), pat dry with a paper towel, and then place on each plate to garnish, along with the chopped chives.

Makes about 5 entrées.

GINGER ORANGE TEMPEH WITH YELLOW WAX BEANS, SWISS CHARD, AND BROWN RICE

For the tempeh:
3 (8-oz.) packages tempeh
2 whole oranges

1 knob peeled fresh ginger (a piece about 1 inch in
    diameter by 3 inches long)
1 cup water
⅔ cup gluten-free tamari or soy sauce

Slice the tempeh across the width on an angle into 1-inch by 2-inch slices.

Grate about 2 tsp. of the rind from the oranges, taking care to avoid the bitter white pith, and save the zest.

Slice the oranges in half.

Slice the ginger into four or five large slices.

Place the tempeh one-layer thick in a large, flat-bottomed pot and add all the other ingredients. Bring to a simmer.

Cook the tempeh for 20 minutes, or until softened.

Remove the tempeh. Strain the cooking liquid and reserve for use in the sauce.

For the wax beans:
1½ tsp. salt
1 lb. fresh wax beans, stem ends removed

Fill a medium stockpot with water and bring to a boil. Add the salt, then add the beans and cook for 8 to 10 minutes, or until softened but still crisp.

Drain the beans and place in a large bowl of ice water to cool and to preserve the green color. Remove from the ice water and set aside.

For the Swiss chard:
¼ cup vegetable oil
2 large bunches roughly chopped Swiss chard or
    other braising greens, stemmed, roughly chopped,
    and washed thoroughly
1 tsp. salt
½ tsp. black pepper

Heat the oil in a large sauté pan and sauté the greens for 5 to 7 minutes, or until slightly wilted (this may be done in batches if necessary).

Season with the salt and pepper and set aside.

To assemble:
1½ Tbsp. arrowroot or cornstarch
1½ Tbsp. cold water
4 cups cooked brown rice (microwavable instant
    works well)
Salt and pepper to taste

Heat the strained liquid from the tempeh in a large braising pan.

In a separate small bowl, stir in the arrowroot and cold water to combine well.

Once the strained liquid reaches a simmer, quickly stir in the cornstarch mixture and cook for 1 minute to thicken.

Add the tempeh and beans and heat through.

Divide the cooked rice among serving plates.

Arrange the heated tempeh, beans, and greens on top of the rice, drizzle sauce on each plate, and serve.

Makes about 5 servings

TAMARI-GLAZED TOFU WRAPS WITH ROASTED PORTOBELLO MUSHROOMS, CORN, AND CHIPOTLE DRESSING

For the tofu:
2 lb. extra-firm tofu
⅓ cup white miso (available at specialty
    Asian markets)
¼ cup olive oil
1 Tbsp. agave nectar
Juice of 2 limes
1 Tbsp. vegetable oil
½ tsp. toasted sesame oil
½ tsp. salt
Cracked black pepper, to taste

Slice the tofu into three or four slices lengthwise, place in a pan with holes or strainer, and press out the water gently with a clean towel.

Press several times and then allow the tofu to drain for 2 to 3 hours.

Slice the blocks into long, thin rectangles of about 3 inches in length and ½ inch cross section.

Mix all the other ingredients well in a bowl. Place the tofu one layer thick on a cookie sheet and pour the marinade on top.

Cook in a preheated 375°F oven for 20 to 25 minutes, turning once, or until the tofu has browned well and the liquid begins to caramelize.

Remove from the oven and cool in the liquid.

For the mushrooms:
5 or 6 large portobello mushrooms
3 Tbsp. olive oil
1 tsp. salt
Cracked black pepper to taste

Remove the stems from the mushrooms. Remove the dark gills from the underside of the mushrooms with a small spoon.

Brush the olive oil evenly over both sides of the mushrooms and place in a single layer on a cookie sheet.

Sprinkle the salt and cracked pepper over both sides of the mushrooms and broil in the oven for 8 to 10 minutes, turning once, or until browned and cooked through.

Remove from the oven. Let cool and then slice into long strips.

For the corn:
5 ears sweet corn (1 (8 to 10-oz.) package frozen corn
    kernels, thawed, unroasted, may be substituted)

Preheat the oven to 425°F, line an oven rack with foil, and place the ears, still in their husks, on the rack. Roast for 35 minutes, or until the kernels have softened.

Remove from the oven and let cool, then remove the husks and silk.

Carefully cut the kernels off each cob with a sharp knife and reserve.

For the chipotle dressing:
1 cup vegan mayonnaise (try Vegenaise)
1½ tsp. chipotle powder
2 tsp. lime juice
½ tsp. salt

Combine all the ingredients well to create a smooth, creamy dressing.

For the wraps:
10 gluten-free tortillas (try Food for Life brand)
3 cups shredded romaine lettuce
3 medium tomatoes, sliced thinly

Toast each tortilla in a dry sauté pan for 2 minutes on each side.

Slather 1 Tbsp. of the chipotle dressing on one side of each tortilla.

Distribute the mushrooms, corn, lettuce, and tomatoes evenly among the wraps and roll into burrito-shaped tubes.

Slice each on an angle through the middle into two halves and serve.

Makes about 10 wraps.

GREEN CURRY COCONUT TEMPEH WITH ASPARAGUS, SWEET PEPPERS, BABY SPINACH, AND BABY BLISS POTATOES

For the tempeh:

3 (8 oz.) packages tempeh

5 cups low-sodium vegetable stock (Pacific Organic
   is a gluten-free, low-sodium option)

2 cups water

1 small knob fresh ginger, peeled, and sliced into
   thin round slices

4 sprigs fresh thyme

2 bay leaves

1 tsp. whole black peppercorns

Slice the tempeh on an angle across the width to create ¾-inch by 1½-inch slices.

Place in a large sauté pan with all the other ingredients, making sure that the tempeh pieces are in a single layer and that the liquid covers all the pieces. Bring to a simmer and cook for 20 minutes, or until softened.

Remove the tempeh and set aside, reserving the liquid and the solids for the sauce.

For the asparagus:

2 bunches thin green asparagus

1½ tsp. salt

Remove the tough ends of the asparagus (cut off about ¼ of the length).

Slice the asparagus into 1 inch slices.

Add the salt to a pot of boiling water, add the asparagus, and blanch for about 3 minutes, or until beginning to soften but still bright green.

Strain and immediately plunge the segments into a bowl full of ice water to cool.

Let cool for 3 minutes, then remove and allow to dry.

For the potatoes:

3 lb. baby red-bliss potatoes, washed well and
    sliced into 1-inch chunks

1½ tsp. salt

Put the potatoes and salt in a pot and cover with 2 inches of water.

Bring to a simmer and cook the potatoes for 15 minutes, or until just tender.

Strain and set aside.

For the sauce:

2¼ cups unsweetened coconut milk

5 Tbsp. Thai green-curry paste

1½ Tbsp. arrowroot

1½ Tbsp. cold water

1 tsp. salt

Combine all the tempeh cooking liquid and solids with the coconut milk and curry paste and bring to a simmer. Cook for 15 minutes, or until the liquid has reduced by a quarter.

Combine the arrowroot and cold water to form a thick paste. Whisk into the simmering liquid and cook for 3 minutes to thicken (more of the arrowroot paste may be necessary if the sauce is too thin, and more water may be added if the sauce becomes too thick).

Season with salt and reserve.

To assemble:

2 red peppers, seeded and cut into strips
2 yellow peppers, seeded and cut into strips
2 Tbsp. vegetable oil
2 cloves garlic, minced
1 tsp. minced ginger
⅔ lb. fairly loosely packed baby spinach
1 tsp. freshly ground black pepper, or to taste
½ tsp. salt, or to taste

Quickly sauté the pepper strips in the oil over medium-high heat for 2 minutes, or until just softened.

Add the garlic and ginger and cook for 1 minute longer.

Add the potatoes, tempeh, and asparagus and heat through.

Strain the sauce into the pan through a fine strainer to allow only the creamy liquid into the pan and heat to simmering.

Add the spinach, cook until barely wilted, and then season with pepper and salt and serve immediately.

Makes 8 servings.

PESTO-ROASTED TOFU OVER ORANGE-SCENTED WHITE BEANS AND GREENS WITH BROILED PEPPERS AND SQUASH

For the beans:

1 qt. dry white beans, cleaned

2 Tbsp. vegetable oil

1 medium onion, diced

2 cloves garlic, minced

1 large orange

2 bay leaves

2 tsp. smoked paprika (regular paprika may be substituted)

2 tsp. freshly ground black pepper

2 sprigs fresh thyme

1½ quarts water

2 bunches roughly chopped braising greens (any varietal will work: Swiss chard, spinach, tatsoi, collard, mustard, etc.)

2 Tbsp. sea salt

2 Tbsp. vegan butter (try Earth Balance brand)

½ tsp. aged sherry vinegar (red-wine vinegar may be substituted)

Place the beans in a large container and add enough cold water to cover by about 4 inches.

Cover and place in the refrigerator overnight. (Note: An alternate method is to soak the beans in very hot water for 2 hours.)

The next day, drain the beans and reserve for cooking.

Heat the oil in a pot and cook the onion for 8 minutes, or until softened.

Add the garlic and cook for another minute.

Grate the whole orange on the finest side of a box grater to remove about 1 Tbsp. orange zest, being careful not to include any of the white pith.

Add the zest, along with the bay leaves, paprika, pepper, thyme, and the soaked beans.

Add enough water to cover the beans, plus about 3 inches, or approximately 1½ quarts.

Cut the orange in half, juice into the pot, and discard the spent halves.

Bring to a simmer and cook for 1½ hours, or until the beans have softened.

Add the greens to the pot and gently wilt for 5 minutes.

Drain most of the excess liquid and season with the salt. Add the "butter" to the beans, then add the vinegar at the very end to brighten the flavor.

For the tofu:
3 lb. extra-firm tofu
3 Tbsp. olive oil
1 tsp. ground cumin
¼ tsp. cayenne pepper
1¼ tsp. sea salt

Drain the tofu well, then turn each block on its side and cut in half, then in half again to create a total of twelve flat planks.

Place the tofu one layer thick into a strainer and gently push down with a clean towel to completely drain the water. Let sit in the refrigerator for 2 hours.

Remove from the strainer and slice each plank into 6 long, rectangular pieces. Combine the remaining ingredients, except the salt, in a bowl and mix well.

Coat the tofu pieces well with the mixture, then place on a cookie sheet one layer thick and season with the salt.

Bake in a 375°F oven for 20 to 25 minutes, or until well browned, turning once. Remove and leave on the cooking sheet; briefly reheat just prior to serving.

For the peppers and squash:
2 whole red bell peppers
2 whole green bell peppers
2 whole yellow or orange bell peppers
3 zucchini squash
3 yellow squash
3 Tbsp. olive oil
2 cloves garlic, minced
1 tsp. sea salt
Freshly cracked black pepper to taste

Cut each pepper into four equal segments, remove the seeds and stems, and place on a cookie sheet.

Slice the squashes into ¼ inch slices at a slight angle down the length to form long, oval slices.

Place the squash slices one layer thick on the cookie sheet with the peppers.

Combine the remaining ingredients, except the pepper, and mix well in a small bowl.

Brush the vegetables well on both sides with the mixture, then crack fresh pepper lightly over both sides. Broil in the oven very close to the heat for about 7 minutes, or until well browned and just softened, turning once.

For the pesto:
½ cup pine nuts
Juice of 2 lemons
2 cloves garlic
½ large bunch flat Italian parsley, washed well
2 large bunches fresh basil, leaves picked from
    the stems
⅔ cup extra-virgin olive oil
1 tsp. sea salt
½ tsp. freshly cracked black pepper, or to taste

Place the nuts, lemon juice, and garlic in a food processor and pulse 7 to 8 times to form a very coarse mixture.

Slice the largest part of the parsley stems off, leaving most of the smaller stems intact.

Add the parsley and basil to the processor and pulse six times, then add the oil slowly during another five to six pulses to form a coarse, bright green pesto.

Season with the salt and pepper and toss the warm tofu pieces in the pesto just prior to serving.

Divide the beans among 8 serving plates. Top with the tofu and arrange the broiled peppers and squash around each plate.

Makes approximately 8 servings.

AUTUMN ROOT VEGETABLE STEW WITH GLAZED TOFU AND GREENS

For the broth:

2½ qt. vegan mushroom broth (try Pacific Natural brand)

½ cup dried porcini or other dried mushrooms

3 bay leaves

4 sprigs fresh thyme

Freshly cracked pepper to taste

Place all the ingredients in a stockpot and simmer for 20 minutes, or until the mushrooms have softened. Remove the thyme sprigs and reserve the broth.

For the tofu:

1½ lb. extra-firm tofu, drained well

½ cup gluten-free tamari

1½ Tbsp. olive oil

1 Tbsp. agave nectar

2 tsp. aged balsamic vinegar

Cut the drained tofu through the length of the block to create ½-inch-thick slabs. Place between two clean kitchen towels and gently press to remove excess water. Cut into ½-inch rough dice.

Combine the remaining ingredients in a large mixing bowl and whisk together.

Toss the tofu in the mixture to coat well.

Place the marinated tofu one layer thick on a cookie sheet and pour the excess marinade on top.

Broil near the oven broiler for 15 to 20 minutes, stirring a few times, or until the tofu is well browned and the marinade is mostly evaporated.

Remove and reserve.

For the stew:

⅓ cup vegetable oil

6 ribs celery, cut into a rough ½-inch dice

4 medium carrots, peeled and cut into a rough ½-inch dice

4 medium turnips, peeled and cut into a rough ½-inch dice

4 medium parsnips, peeled and cut into a rough ½-inch dice*

1 medium onion, chopped

1¾ lb. cremini mushrooms, stems removed and halved

5 cloves garlic, chopped

¼ cup aged balsamic vinegar

2 (14.5-oz.) cans diced tomatoes

1 lb. baby red bliss potatoes, washed and cut into quarters

2 Tbsp. chopped fresh rosemary
2 bunches dark green braising greens (turnip,
    collard, mustard, Swiss chard, or any
    combination), washed well and chopped
Salt and cracked black pepper to taste

Heat the oil in a large stockpot on high heat for 1 minute.

Carefully add the celery, carrots, turnips, and parsnips and sauté on high heat for 5 minutes, stirring often to prevent sticking.

Add the onion and cook over medium-high heat for 3 minutes longer.

Add the mushrooms and cook for another 7 to 8 minutes, or until the mushrooms and vegetables begin to soften.

Add the garlic and cook for an additional minute.

Place the vinegar in the pot and cook until the liquid is nearly evaporated and the mixture takes on a deep-brown color.

Add the tomatoes, potatoes, reserved broth, and rosemary and simmer for 15 to 20 minutes, or until the potatoes just begin to soften.

Add the greens and simmer gently to wilt, about 2 to 3 minutes.

Add the tofu, stir well to combine, and season with salt and cracked pepper, being careful not to over season since the mushroom broth is presalted.

Note: Any hard root vegetables may be substituted for the ones listed above.

Makes about 10 servings.

SIDES

Hearty Greens with Pecans and Olives

4 Tbsp. olive oil
2 qt. chopped Swiss chard
2 qt. chopped turnip greens
1 cup chopped black olives
½ cup pecan pieces
¼ cup capers, drained
3 Tbsp. chopped garlic
Juice of 1 lemon
1 tsp. sea salt
Cracked black pepper to taste

Heat the oil in a large sauté or braising pan.

Add the greens and cook over high heat for 3 to 5 minutes, or until wilted and softened.

Add the olives, pecans, capers, and garlic, and cook for an additional minute.

Add the lemon juice and season with the salt and pepper.

Makes 8 sides.

STEAMED BABY BOK CHOY WITH
AGAVE ORANGE GLAZE

For the bok choy:
1½ lb. baby bok choy, washed well
1 tsp. salt

Cut each bok choy in half.

Add the salt to a pot full of water, bring to a simmer, add the bok choy and cook in the salted water for 3 to 5 minutes, or until just tender.

Remove and immediately plunge into a bowl of ice water to cool completely and preserve the green color.

Drain very well once cooled.

To assemble:
1 ripe orange
¼ cup dark amber agave nectar
½ tsp. powdered ginger
½ tsp. salt
Cooked boy choy from above
2 Tbsp. vegan butter (try Earth Balance brand)
Salt and pepper to taste

Using the finest holes of a box grater, rasp about 1 tsp. of the orange skin from the outside of the orange, avoiding the bitter white pith.

Juice the orange, strain to remove the seeds, and place in a small saucepan with the grated zest, agave, ginger, and salt.

Simmer for 10 minutes, or until reduced by two-thirds and syrupy.

Place the bok choy and glaze in a large skillet and heat for about 1 minute or until heated through.

Swirl in the vegan butter to create a creamy glaze.

Season with salt and pepper.

Makes about 5 servings.

ROASTED BEETS AND GOLD POTATOES

For the beets:

5 medium beets

5 whole, peeled garlic cloves

5 sprigs fresh thyme

1 Tbsp. whole black peppercorns

1 Tbsp. sea salt

1¼ cup olive oil

Slice off the root ends and tops of the beets and wash well in cold water.

Toss the beets with all the other ingredients to coat well.

Place in a single layer in a baking dish, cover with foil, and roast in a 375°F oven for 45 minutes, or until tender.

Remove from the oven, let cool, and cut beets into 1-inch dice.

For the potatoes:

1 lb. baby gold potatoes (large gold or baby red bliss may be substituted)

3 Tbsp. olive oil

2 tsp. chopped rosemary
Salt and black pepper to taste

Thoroughly wash the potatoes in cold water and drain well.

Slice the potatoes in half or in quarters, if they are large, to form a large dice.

Toss the potatoes in the oil, add the rosemary, and season lightly with the salt and pepper.

Place in a single layer on a baking sheet and roast in a 425°F oven for 25 to 30 minutes, stirring once, or until well browned and softened.

Combine with the beets and garlic and serve.

Makes about 8 servings.

ROASTED AUTUMN ROOT VEGETABLES

1 lb. carrots, peeled
1 lb. sweet potatoes or yams, washed well
1 lb. turnips, peeled
1 lb. gold potatoes, washed well
¼ cup olive oil
¼ cup chopped fresh parsley
2 Tbsp. chopped fresh rosemary
2 Tbsp. chopped garlic
1½ Tbsp. salt
1 Tbsp. chopped fresh thyme
Cracked black pepper, to taste

Cut all the vegetables into a large, rough dice, approximately 1 inch square.

Toss with all the other ingredients in a large bowl to coat the vegetables well.

Place in a single layer on baking sheets and roast in a 425°F oven for 25 minutes, stirring once or twice, or until well browned and softened.

Makes about 8 servings.

GINGER GREENS WITH SHIITAKE MUSHROOMS

For the greens:
2 Tbsp. olive oil
1 cup sliced shiitake mushrooms, stems removed
1 lb. braising greens (try tatsoi, kale, chard, spinach, or beet), washed very well and coarsely chopped
1½ Tbsp. minced fresh ginger
2 Tbsp. soy sauce
1½ tsp. rice-wine vinegar
Salt and cracked black pepper to taste

Heat the olive oil in a large skillet, add the mushrooms, and cook over medium-high heat for 5 minutes.

Add the greens and ginger and cook for an additional 3 minutes, or until the greens wilt.

Add the remaining ingredients and mix well.

Season with salt and pepper.

Makes about 5 servings.

LEMON-PEPPER BROCCOLI

1 head of broccoli
2 Tbsp. vegan butter (try Earth Balance brand)

1 clove garlic, minced
Juice of ½ lemon
1 tsp. coarse black pepper

Remove the stem from the broccoli and cut the florets into bite-size pieces.

Bring an inch of water to a boil in a saucepan. Place the broccoli in a steamer basket, cover with a lid, and place over the saucepan. Cook for 4 to 5 minutes, so that the broccoli is still slightly crisp. Remove from the heat and drain.

In a sauté pan, melt the vegan butter over medium heat, add the garlic, and cook for 45 seconds.

Stir in the lemon juice and pepper, then add the broccoli and stir again. Cook for 1 to 2 minutes, or until the desired consistency is reached.

Makes 2 to 4 servings.

SESAME-GRILLED ASPARAGUS

1 lb. fresh asparagus, trimmed
2 Tbsp. sesame oil
Salt and pepper to taste
2 Tbsp. toasted sesame seeds

Preheat a grill or grill pan to medium heat.

Coat the asparagus with the sesame oil by tossing or brushing, then sprinkle with salt and pepper.

Place on the grill and cook for 4 to 5 minutes, turning every minute or so.

Remove from the heat and sprinkle with sesame seeds.

Makes 4 servings.

DESSERTS

Strawberry Lemonade Granita

1 cup cold water
½ cup lemon juice
½ cup agave nectar
4½ cups hulled organic strawberries

In a blender or food processor, combine the water, lemon juice, and agave nectar and blend. Pulse three to four times and then puree.

Add half the strawberries and purée the mixture until smooth. Add the remaining berries and purée until completely smooth.

Pour the liquid mixture into a shallow plastic freezer container about 8 by 10 inches. Place in the freezer for about 45 minutes, or until the edges become icy.

Using a fork, stir the ice into the center and return the pan to the freezer. Repeat the stirring every 40 minutes, or until solid, about 6 hours.

Once solid, use a fork to scrape down the solid mixture to create flakes. Repeat until the entire mixture is flaky. Cover and freeze.

Makes 4 servings.

APPLE PIE

For the crust:

1½ cups rice flour

½ tsp. salt

1 tsp. xanthan gum

⅓ cup vegan butter, chilled (try Earth Balance brand)

⅓ cup vegetable shortening, chilled

¼ cup cold water

Preheat the oven to 350°F.

Put the rice flour, salt, and xanthan gum into the bowl of a food processor and blend until well combined.

Either by hand or in the food processor, cut in chunks of the "butter" and shortening.

Add the water a little at a time until a ball is formed, being careful not to overmix. Divide the dough into two equal-size balls. Wrap tightly in plastic and refigerate for one hour.

Roll the dough to ⅛ inch thickness. Invert one sheet of dough onto a 9-inch pie pan. Reserve the other sheet of dough.

Prick the piecrust with a fork. Bake for 15 minutes, until brown.

For the filling:

1¾ lb. Golden Delicious apples, cored, peeled, and thinly sliced

1¾ lb. Granny Smith apples, cored, peeled, and thinly sliced

¼ cup agave nectar

1 tsp. fresh lemon juice

½ tsp. vanilla extract

½ tsp. ground cinnamon

1 Tbsp. rice flour

Preheat the oven to 400°F.

In a large bowl, combine the apples, agave, lemon juice, vanilla extract, and cinnamon. Let stand for approximately 15 minutes, or until juices form. Add the flour and mix.

To assemble:

Soy milk

Spoon the filling into the bottom of the prebaked crust. Drape the second sheet of dough over the filling.

Seal the top and bottom crust edges together and trim any excess dough, leaving a ½-inch overhang. Fold under and crimp decoratively with a greased fork.

Brush the pie with the soy milk.

Transfer to a baking sheet and place in the oven.

Immediately reduce the temperature to 375°F. Bake for approximately 2 hours, or until the crust is golden brown, the apples are tender, and the filling is thick and bubbling. If the edges are browning too quickly, cover with foil.

Makes 8 servings.

CHOCOLATE RASPBERRY MOUSSE PIE

For the dough:

¾ cup rice flour

¼ tsp. salt

½ tsp. xanthan gum

2 Tbsp. + 1 tsp. vegan butter, chilled (try Earth Balance brand)

2 Tbsp. + 1 tsp. vegetable shortening, chilled
2 Tbsp. cold water

Preheat the oven to 350°F.

Put the rice flour, salt, and xanthan gum in the bowl of a food processor and blend until well combined.

Either by hand or in the food processor, cut in chunks of the vegan butter and shortening.

Add the water a little at a time until a ball is formed, being careful not to overmix.

Roll the dough to a ⅛-inch thickness and invert onto a 9-inch pie pan. Trim the overhanging edges.

Prick the dough with a fork and bake for 15 minutes, until brown.

For the filling:
1¼ lb. silken tofu (2½ packages)
¾ cup agave nectar
¼ cup soy milk
1 Tbsp. vanilla
⅔ cup high-quality unsweetened cocoa powder
¼ cup raspberries (plus more for garnish)

Mix the tofu in a food processor for several minutes, until very smooth. Add the agave nectar, soy milk, and vanilla. Pulse once or twice to blend. Add the cocoa and raspberries and blend until smooth. Fill the baked crust with the tofu mixture and chill until slightly firm.

Garnish with additional raspberries and serve.

Makes 8 servings.

WHERE TO FIND PRODUCTS
USED ON THE CLEANSE

GLUTEN-FREE WEBSITES AND RESOURCES

GlutenFree.com: http://www.glutenfree.com/

The Gluten-Free Mall: http://www.glutenfreemall.com/

Gluten-Free Trading Company: http://www.food4 celiacs.com/

GLUTEN-FREE BREADS AND CRACKERS

Gluten-Free Bakehouse (Whole Foods gluten-free line): http://www.wholefoodsmarket.com/products/ gluten-free-products.php

Edward and Sons Rice Snaps: http://www.edward andsons.com/es_shop_snaps.itml

Bob's Red Mill bread and pancake mixes: http:// www.bobsredmill.com/home.php?cat=126

Kinnikinnick bread and crackers: http://www. kinnikinnick.com/

Glutino bread and crackers: http://www.glutino.com/ content/view/53/62/

Ener-G bread and crackers: http://www.ener-g.com/

Food for Life bread: http://foodforlife.com/
  gluten-free-wheat-free-breads.html

Blue Diamond Nut-Thins crackers: http://www.blue
  diamond.com/shop/natural/nutThins.cfm

Mary's Gone Crackers: http://www.marysgonecrackers
  .com

VEGAN, NATURALLY SWEETENED ENERGY/PROTEIN BARS

Lärabars: http://www.larabar.com

PranaBars: http://www.pranabars.com/

VEGA Bars: http://sequelnaturals.com/vega

Organic Food Bar http://www.organicfoodbar.com/

VEGAN MAYONNAISE

Spectrum Light Canola Mayo: http://www.spectrum
  organics.com/?id=57#j204

Follow Your Heart Veganaise: http://www.followyour
  heart.com/vegenaise.html

Nayonaise: http://www.nasoya.com/nasoya/nayonaise
  _index.html

VEGAN BUTTER

Earth Balance and Soy Garden: http://www.earth
  balancenatural.com/#/products/

Spectrum Organics Spectrum Spread: http://www
  .spectrumorganics.com/?id=57#j124

PROTEIN POWDERS

Solaray Soytein Powder: www.allstarhealth.com/f/
  solaray-soytein_soy_protein-powder.htm

NutriBiotic Rice Protein Powder: http://www.nutri
biotic.com/rice-protein.html

HELP WITH VEGAN FOOD
VegAdvantage: http://www.vegadvantage.com/

HEALTH AND NUTRITION RESOURCES
Physicians Committee for Responsible Medicine:
http://pcrm.org/
Nutrition MD: http://www.nutritionmd.org

ANIMAL PROTECTION WEBSITES
The Humane Society of the United States: http://
www.hsus.org
Farm Sanctuary: http://farmsanctuary.org
People for the Ethical Treatment of Animals: http://
www.peta.org

QUICKIE MEALS AND SNACKS

IF YOU DON'T HAVE TIME TO COOK UP A FULL MEAL, I'VE IN-
cluded a list of "quickies" that can be thrown together easily in a pinch. You will find your own favorites, too, the more
you get used to the cleanse.

BREAKFAST

Rice cakes or toasted gluten-free bread with almond
or peanut butter.

Soy yogurt mixed with 2 tablespoons flaxseed oil, almonds, and chopped apples, pears, or blueberries.

Any kind of hot, whole-grain, unprocessed cereal
(other than wheat-based ones) sprinkled with
chopped nuts and apples, with rice, hemp, soy, or
almond milk poured on top.

Toasted frozen gluten-free waffles topped with vegan
butter and drizzled with agave nectar.

Gluten-free bagel with vegan cream cheese, vegan
butter, or nut butter.

Leftover brown rice (or almost any cooked grain)—
hot or cold—with nuts and blueberries, non-dairy
milk poured over.

LUNCH

Any vegan canned or deli soup (homemade is even
better!) with vegetables and/or beans as a base.
Lentil, black bean, minestrone, squash, gazpa-
cho, etc.

Kitchen-sink salad. Throw in anything you can find
in your kitchen, such as veggies, seeds, dried
cranberries, avocado, etc. Top with veggie burger,
crumbled tempeh, or baked tofu.

Taco shell or corn tortilla with black beans, avocado,
lettuce, salsa, and vegan sour cream.

Sandwich with thinly sliced tempeh or crumbled
tofu, scallions, vegan mayonnaise, sliced tomato,
avocado, onion, and mustard.

Nori (seaweed) paper wrapped around sprouts,
cucumber, avocado, and long cuts of baked tofu
with rice.

A smoothie made with vegan protein powder, coconut
or regular water, a few cubes of ice, 2 tablespoons
freshly ground flaxseed, 2 tablespoons flax oil, a
small handful of raw almonds, walnuts, or hemp
seeds, a handful of blueberries (optional), and a cup
and a half of frozen broccoli, spinach, or cauliflower.
(Trust me, you won't taste the vegetables. This
one's great as a protein boost after exercise, too!)

SNACKS

Sliced apples with nut butter.

Bowl of blueberries with soy creamer poured over them.

Fruit salad.

Small handful of nuts or seeds.

Small handful of goji berries (mixed with nuts is even better!).

Guacamole, salsa, and corn chips.

Hummus and cucumbers, carrots, or chips.

Powdered green drink (there are many varieties available on the Web and in health food stores) blended with either water or 3 ounces of apple juice and 3 ounces of water.

DINNER

Baked sweet potato (microwave if you must) with sautéed or steamed vegetables (kale or broccoli is great) and grilled tofu. Use olive oil, garlic, and salt to taste, or a favorite bottled sauce. You might also cube the potato and roast it if you don't want to wait for it to bake!

Shredded spaghetti squash (it looks like pasta!). Just cut in half lengthwise, bake, and use a fork to shred the inside. Toss with olive oil and salt or jarred pasta sauce with sautéed tofu on the side.

Kitchen-sink salad (see "Lunch").

Stir-fried veggies and tempeh or tofu over a bed of brown rice or quinoa.

Mediterranean platter with hummus, cucumbers, baba ghanoush (mashed eggplant), and flax or gluten-free crackers or bread.

Simple rice and beans with veggies (use frozen vegetables if you don't have time, but fresh is better).

DESSERTS

Herbal tea with or without soy creamer.

Fresh fruit with a dollop of soy yogurt and a drizzle of agave nectar (add chopped pistachios for a special treat). Choose fruits that are low on the glycemic index.

ACKNOWLEDGEMENTS

I AM SO OFTEN AWESTRUCK BY HOW THINGS COME TOGETHER AS perfectly as they do, and how I've been graced to make the acquaintance of so many brilliant and generous people. Truly, I am humbled.

My most heartfelt thanks go to:

Everyone at Weinstein Books: Harvey Weinstein, Judy Hottensen, Kristin Powers, Katie Finch, Richard Florest, Danielle Plafsky, and Adrian Palacios. You are the dream team of publishers—passionate, skillful, and talented. I know I am in great hands with you.

Dr. Dean Ornish, who gifted me with his substantial and highly informative foreword; you are a fierce advocate for taking health into our own hands (while showing us how at every step). The medical and wellness community is lucky to have you, and I am so very honored to know you.

Marianne Williamson, the reigning queen of spiritual and self-help gurus; your words and guidance will always ring in my heart. What a true and powerful voice you are.

Tal Ronnen, the genius in the kitchen, who along with Lex Townes, came up with the divine and delicious recipes. You are an inspiration to all of us who are mere mortals in the culinary arts (even though you've made compassionate cooking extremely easy).

Caroline Pincus who is my beloved editor; where would I be without your sharp eye and ability to prune and sculpt a sentence? I shudder to think. How I love working with you!

Dr. Neal Barnard, to whom I have turned countless times for guidance on peer-reviewed studies and a more thorough understanding of how the body works and thrives; you are an agent of change in the health and wellness world, and I'm grateful for your persevering research.

Bruce Friedrich, who is an inspired and brilliant educator and activist for all things animal-related; I am so blessed to know you and work with you. I would never have found the right words without you.

Lisa Lange, a fierce and savvy advocate for animals; you have been a trustworthy and wise adviser. And a wonderful friend.

Jannette Patterson: you gently persuaded me to look at videos and pictures of what happens to animals behind closed doors; you helped to open my eyes with the perfect balance of persistence and patience. What a lovely soul you are.

Wayne Pacelle: I am forever stirred by the way you systematically go about creating a more humane society; from you I have learned to use my life well, and to squeeze every drop from the day. You are a force, my dear friend.

Kevin Law, whose research and writing I am always

deeply impressed by and grateful for. Never mind that you are my brother; you are one of the brightest minds around.

Barry Michels and Phil Stutz, for their keen guidance in all things psychological (and spiritual). Your insights, tools, and exercises should be required learning.

Armand Bytton, for the journeys you've taken me on to know myself better so that I could communicate more effectively. You are sage and shaman.

Jennifer Rudolph Walsh, Jim Wiatt, and everyone at the William Morris Agency; your judicious and warm counsel have kept me steady and well-informed. I am grateful for your sound advice.

Nicki Graham, my assistant and researcher; you are infinitely resourceful in so many different arenas, and I very much appreciate the light you bring to everything you do.

Emily Votruba, for your spot-on copyediting.

Brian Nice, for your fresh and cheerful photography (again).

Brian Chojnowski, for your delightful design.

And most of all, my husband Tom, who has rolled with all the changes I have gone through during our marriage. I know I am not who I was back in the beginning of our time together, and I am forever grateful for how you have allowed (and encouraged) me to grow. Thank you for the doors you've opened in my heart, and for the windows into a greater world you have helped me to see.